Concepts in
DRUG METABOLISM

DRUGS AND THE PHARMACEUTICAL SCIENCES

A Series of Textbooks and Monographs

Edited by

James Swarbrick
School of Pharmacy
University of Southern California
Los Angeles, California

Other Volumes in Preparation

Concepts in
DRUG METABOLISM

(IN TWO PARTS)

Part A

EDITED BY

PETER JENNER
University Department of Neurology
Institute of Psychiatry and
King's College Hospital Medical School
London, England

BERNARD TESTA
Department of Medicinal Chemistry
School of Pharmacy
University of Lausanne
Lausanne, Switzerland

MARCEL DEKKER, INC.   New York and Basel

Library of Congress Cataloging in Publication Data

Main entry under title:

Concepts in drug metabolism.

    (Drugs and the pharmaceutical sciences ; v. 10)
    Includes indexes.
    1. Drug metabolism. I. Jenner, Peter,
[date] II. Testa, Bernard.
RM301.55.C66   615'.7   80-12792
ISBN 0-8247-6906-6

MARCEL DEKKER, INC.
270 Madison Avenue, New York, New York 10016

Current printing (last digit):
10 9 8 7 6 5 4 3 2

PRINTED IN THE UNITED STATES OF AMERICA

PREFACE

The Development of Concepts in Drug Metabolism

    At least a century ago it was recognized that ingested drugs or other
foreign compounds are excreted either unchanged or chemically modified.*
At that time, however, the chemical alteration of drugs by living tissues
was regarded mainly as a curiosity of little importance in terms of main-
stream scientific advances, which saw the establishment of the fundamentals
of modern chemistry, biochemistry, and pharmacology. Although preoc-
cupation with the early development of these three disciplines caused a
neglect of research into drug metabolism per se, ironically the same disciplines were later to provide the basis of its methodology and the foundation
of its principles. Despite the neglect just mentioned, a considerable body
of information was generated during the later part of the nineteenth century
and the beginning of the twentieth century, leading to the initial concept of
drugs undergoing a number of distinct chemical changes within the intact
organism. Truly, many major pathways of drug metabolism that are readily accepted today were first reported during this era.
    What then formed the major advances that have caused the study of
drug metabolism to evolve from its embryonic existence and to distinguish
itself from its parent sciences of chemistry, biochemistry, pharmacology,
and toxicology?
    First, there was a realization that the processes of drug metabolism
might be of importance in determining the pharmacological activity, clinical
efficacy, and toxicological profile of drug molecules. The increased effort
put into the subsequent investigation of drug metabolism processes led to
the emergence of specialists in this area of research. The significance of
this human factor cannot be overestimated, since it is the ultimate limiting
factor in the development of any science, as it is in fact in human progress
generally.
    This realization would have had a comparatively limited impact were
it not for the concurrent improvement that occurred in analytical technology.

----

*A. Conti and M. H. Bickel, Drug Metab. Rev. 6:1 (1977).

iii

Thus, advances in the selectivity, sensitivity, and accuracy of the analytical tools, as well as the development of methods specifically designed for drug metabolism studies, have played a major role in formulating the science of drug metabolism as we understand it.

It was during the 1940s that the work of pioneers such as the late R. T. Williams and B. B. Brodie, whose ideas were far ahead of their time, led to the opening of the road to modern progress.[*] Indeed, it was during this period that the concepts of drug metabolism were extended to establish principles such as Phase I and Phase II metabolism, which remain viable today.

Following this lead a rapid maturation of drug metabolism research occurred in the 1950s, and development has continued exponentially until the present day. In fact, the last two decades have seen the field of drug metabolism gain a reputable status and establish itself as a new science. The importance of drug metabolism and disposition on biological activity has become universally recognized. As a result of stringent legal requirements governing the use of novel drug molecules in humans, many countries have made metabolism studies compulsory. This in turn has done much to increase the amount of energy (both human and financial) applied to the adolescent science.

The increased necessity for such drug metabolism studies has led to a rapid growth in the relevant literature. Indeed, the current flood of data threatens to overwhelm researchers. They must feel the need to walk uphill in search of original approaches and generalizing concepts.[†] This situation presents difficulties and, in our opinion, must only be transitional if drug metabolism is to mature into a full science. The need for unifying concepts exists and is perceived by many, if not yet clearly. For example, a number of reviews and monographs have appeared in recent years that have attempted to bring some semblance of order to drug metabolism or its subfields by classifying and organizing the mass of available data.

We feel the time is now ripe for the members of the drug metabolism community to once again focus on the concepts which govern their science. A concept, the dictionary informs us, is "the idea of the attributes common to a class of things." With this as a goal we have invited a number of our colleagues to undertake an uphill contemplation of an area of drug metabolism research and to present the reader with a wide-ranging and conceptual approach to major topics in drug metabolism and allied fields. This has led to some overlap between contributions—which we have encouraged, since the relationships and interdependence between topics thus become more evident and the confrontation of viewpoints is often provocative and refreshing.

---

[*]L. Young, in Drug Metabolism: From Microbe to Man (D. V. Parke and R. L. Smith, eds.), Taylor & Francis, London, 1977, pp. 1-11.
[†]B. Testa, Drug Metab. Rev. 5(2):i (1976).

Due to the very requirements of the conceptual approach, the various chapters in the present work reflect the personalities and views of their authors more than do ordinary reviews. The reader will find some chapters to be quite philosophical in their approach, whereas others make use of a large body of factual examples to illustrate the underlying concepts. In either case, however, we hope to show how vital is the generation of concepts and generalizing theories if the study of drug metabolism is to become a mature science—a science in which results can be predicted and not guessed, and which can in turn fertilize other sciences through its own discoveries.

Peter Jenner
Bernard Testa

CONTRIBUTORS

LUC P. BALANT, Ph.D. Privat-Docent in Pharmacokinetics, Department of Medicine, University of Geneva, Geneva, Switzerland

JOHN CALDWELL, Ph.D. Senior Lecturer in Biochemical Pharmacology, Department of Biochemical and Experimental Pharmacology, St. Mary's Hospital Medical School, London, England

RONALD T. COUTTS, Ph.D., D.Sc. Professor of Medicinal Chemistry and Assistant Dean, Faculty of Pharmacy and Pharmaceutical Sciences, University of Alberta, Edmonton, Alberta, Canada

EINO HIETANEN, M.D.[*] Senior Lecturer in Physiology, Department of Physiology, University of Kuopio, Kuopio, Finland

PETER JENNER, Ph.D., M.P.S. Senior Lecturer in Biochemistry, University Department of Neurology, Institute of Psychiatry and King's College Hospital Medical School, London, England

GRAHAM R. JONES, Ph.D.[†] Research Associate, Faculty of Pharmacy and Pharmaceutical Sciences, University of Alberta, Edmonton, Alberta, Canada

JAMES McAINSH, M.Sc., Ph.D. Senior Investigator, Department of Safety of Medicines, Imperial Chemical Industries Limited, Pharmaceuticals Division, Macclesfield, England

---

Present affiliations:
[*]Acting Professor, Department of Physiology, University of Turku, Turku, Finland
[†]Senior Laboratory Scientist, Department of Laboratory Medicine, University of Alberta Hospital, Edmonton, Alberta, Canada

OLAVI PELKONEN, M.D.   Acting Associate Professor, Department of
Pharmacology, University of Oulu, Oulu, Finland

BERNARD TESTA, Ph.D.   Professor and Chairman of Medicinal Chemistry, Department of Medicinal Chemistry, School of Pharmacy, University
of Lausanne, Lausanne, Switzerland

WILLIAM F. TRAGER, Ph.D.   Professor of Pharmaceutical Chemistry,
Department of Pharmaceutical Sciences, University of Washington, Seattle,
Washington

HARRY VAINIO, M.D.   Chief, Department of Industrial Hygiene and
Toxicology, Institute of Occupational Health, Helsinki, Finland

CONTENTS

CONTENTS OF PART B

Chapter 1

SIGNIFICANCE OF ANALYTICAL TECHNIQUES IN DRUG METABOLISM STUDIES

Ronald T. Coutts and Graham R. Jones[*]

Faculty of Pharmacy and Pharmaceutical Sciences
University of Alberta
Edmonton, Alberta, Canada

The four major steps in most drug metabolism studies are the isolation of a given drug and its metabolites from biological media, the separation of the components that have been isolated, the identification of each component, and the quantification of recovered drug and metabolites. These four steps are considered in the present chapter, which examines extractive procedures (solvents, resins, charcoal) as used for isolation purposes, chromatographic techniques (GC, HPLC, TLC) allowing separation, spectroscopic methods (UV, IR, NMR, MS) allowing identification, and several quantitative methods (GC, HPLC, mass fragmentography).

When discussing these methods and techniques, the emphasis is laid on their applicability to drug metabolism studies, on their advantages and limitations in influencing the design of such studies, and on their significance in determining the value and reliability of drug metabolism data.

---

[*]Present affiliation: Department of Laboratory Medicine, University of Alberta Hospital, Edmonton, Alberta, Canada.

I. INTRODUCTION

Interest in the metabolism of drugs and xenobiotics has greatly increased
during the last two decades. A major reason for this is undoubtedly the
current availability of sensitive, specific, and reproducible methods of isolating, separating, identifying, and quantifying small quantities of organic
compounds. Drug metabolism studies are conducted by pharmacologists,
biochemists, organic, analytical, and pharmaceutical chemists and by per-
sonnel in other scientific disciplines, each of whom emphasizes different
aspects of metabolism. Globally however, the investigator is required to
isolate the drug and its metabolites from biological tissues or fluids, separate
the components that have been isolated, identify each component, and in
many instances quantify the amounts of recovered drug and each metabolite
isolated.

The diversity of interest in the subject, and the volume of published
material, preclude the possibility of examining all the techniques of interest
in drug metabolism studies; only those which are employed often or which
are of value in particular instances are described. Excluded from consideration in this chapter is the important technique of radiolabeling. Also,
the stereochemical methodology is scarcely considered, and the interested
reader is referred to a recent review of the subject by Testa and Jenner [1].

In most instances, urine and blood (or plasma) are the biological fluids
which are investigated for drugs and metabolites. Other materials, including breast milk, bile, saliva, cerebrospinal fluid, eye fluids, perspira-
tion, as well as feces, may be analyzed—but not routinely. Tissues, especially brain, liver, kidney and lung, are occasionally examined in animal
distribution and metabolism studies.

II. ISOLATION PROCEDURES

Various procedures are employed to isolate drugs and metabolites from
biological samples. The two most common are solvent extraction and the
use of resins and adsorbents.

A. Solvent Extraction

  1. Choice of Apparatus

  Removal of organic compounds from biological solutions or tissue homogenates most often involves extraction with suitable water-immiscible organic solvents after the pH of the biological sample has been adjusted to an appropriate value. If small volumes of biological samples are to be extracted, mechanical rocking shakers [e.g., the Aliquot Mixer (Ames Co.)] or vortex mixers [e.g., the Vortex-Genie mixer (Scientific Industries Inc.)] are convenient. If relatively large volumes have to be extracted, conventional separatory funnels or continuous extractors (available from Sargent-Welch Scientific Co.) are employed. The latter are available in two types, which permits the use of solvents with densities lower or higher than the aqueous layer being investigated.

  2. Concentration of Sample

  When large volumes of urine or other biological fluids are investigated, it is sometimes necessary to concentrate the sample prior to solvent extraction. The use of heat should be avoided, since labile compounds may be destroyed and volatile compounds lost at elevated temperatures. Evaporation under reduced pressure, and freeze-drying (lyophilization) are suitable methods. Hucker et al. [1a] employed an interesting technique which resulted in a 25-fold concentration of a large urine sample. The urine was saturated with anhydrous sodium sulfate and extracted with isopropanol. Evaporation of the isopropanol gave the concentrated aqueous residue.

  3. Choice of Solvent

  In extraction procedures, the choice of solvent is often an arbitrary one. Solvents which are commonly employed are chloroform, diethyl ether, ethyl acetate, methylene chloride, benzene, toluene, and isopropanol, or mixtures of them. Isopropyl chloride is not often used in extraction procedures, but consideration of its properties (BP 36°; dielectric constant 9.82; water solubility 1.3%) suggests that it might be an excellent solvent which should be used more often [2]. Solvents should be distilled immediately prior to use so as to ensure that they are free of trace quantities of solutes, which could interfere with subsequent analyses. Phthalates, for example, are ubiquitous, and some solvents, especially diethyl ether, may contain antioxidants such as butylated hydroxytoluene (BHT) that could be erroneously identified as metabolites. Traces of peroxides also form rapidly in diethyl ether samples and can convert drugs and metabolites to oxygenated products which may be erroneously identified as additional metabolites.

4. Extraction Procedures

Since drugs and metabolites may be neutral, acidic, basic, or amphoteric compounds, it is necessary to adjust the pH of the solution which is
being extracted to effect as complete an extraction as possible. Such a
procedure is not without its disadvantages. Some drugs or metabolites are
labile compounds and sensitive to changes in pH. Chemical degradations
may occur during the extraction procedures, and products of such degradations can easily be mistakenly identified as metabolites. If the substrate is
a neutral compound or an acidic drug, chemical degradations occur less
frequently than with basic substrates. The majority of metabolites formed
from neutral or acidic drugs are C-oxygenated products, especially phenols,
carboxylic acids, ketones, and aldehydes, which are relatively easy to isolate from neutralized or acidified solutions with many organic solvents, so
that good-to-excellent recoveries of drugs and metabolites are usually possible. If, however, the substrate is a basic compound, a variety of metabolites (basic, neutral, acidic, and amphoteric) is possible. A common practice is to adjust the pH of the solution successively to 12.0, 8.5-9.5, and
1.0 and extract with a suitable solvent at each of these pH values. Such a
procedure will extract, respectively, stable basic and neutral compounds,
amphoteric products, and acidic compounds. Sulfates and other water-
soluble drug conjugates are not extracted by such a procedure, and the extraction of glucuronides and amphoteric compounds is rarely complete. In
addition, many primary N-oxygenated metabolites of basic drugs and chemicals are sensitive to changes in pH and undergo isomerism or chemical
degradation during extraction procedures [3].

A major disadvantage of solvent extraction procedures is that, regardless of the pH to which the solution has been adjusted, some drugs and metabolites (e.g., sulfate conjugates) cannot be extracted with solvents from
aqueous solutions. If metabolites are present in conjugate form, it is often
the practice to hydrolyze an aliquot of the biological solution with an enzyme
preparation (β-glucuronidase and sulfatase) or with hot mineral acid prior
to extraction. Both processes liberate metabolites from their conjugates,
and these metabolites can then be removed from aqueous solution by conventional solvent extraction techniques. Sulfates can also be isolated from
aqueous solution by means of an anion exchange column [4].

Some drugs and metabolites become firmly bound to protein in the
biological system. In these instances the addition of trichloroacetic acid
(a protein precipitant) or other reagents may be of value, but such treatment may result in the decomposition of acid-labile metabolites. One advantage of investigating urine samples for drug metabolites is that urine
is normally devoid of protein.

5. Extraction Efficiency

The solvent extraction method used to remove drugs and metabolites
from biological fluids should be the most efficient one possible. In practice,

however, decisions on how many extractions to make or on how long to continue a continuous extraction are often made arbitrarily. If the identity of
the metabolite is known, the biological sample can be "spiked" with a small
amount of an authentic sample of the metabolite and the amount of it removed
by the extraction method chosen can be ascertained (see section on quantitative analysis). Alternatively, if a [14]C- or ^{3}H-labeled sample of authentic
metabolite is available, then the efficiency of the chosen method is easily
established by adding trace amounts of the radioactive compound to aliquots
of the solution being extracted and continuing the extraction procedure until
the aqueous layer is devoid of radioactivity.

In many instances, however, the identities of metabolites are not known
and extraction efficiency is difficult to ascertain.

6. Ion-Pair Extraction

The technique of ion-pair extraction can be used to remove hydrophilic,
ionizable compounds from aqueous solution. This is often difficult to do
using conventional liquid-liquid extraction. By careful selection of the
counterion required to form a strong ion pair with the sample ion, a lipophilic ion pair will result that may be extracted in good yield into a suitable
solvent. Morphine and bromothymol, for example, form a strong ion pair
which is extractable from aqueous solution into methylene chloride [5]. The
method may be used to remove both hydrophilic drugs and metabolites from
biological fluids, although a single counterion may not be ideal for pairing
with all the metabolites present.

Ion pairs can be chromatographed without dissociation by thin layer
chromatography (TLC) or high pressure liquid chromatography (HPLC).
HPLC separations of several biogenic amines and some of their metabolites
have been described [6]. Alternatively, the extract of ion pairs may be
analyzed by gas chromatography (GC); the complexes usually dissociate in
the injection port or on-column, particularly if the stationary phase is ap-
propriately chosen. For example, a base-sulfonic acid ion pair would dissociate, and the base would chromatograph on an alkaline GC column [7].

Hydrophilic anions such as glucuronides and amino acids have been
extracted from aqueous solutions by forming ion pairs with large quaternary
ammonium ions [8,9], although the technique is currently little used in
metabolism studies. Catecholamines have been extracted from aqueous
solutions in excellent yield by the use of adduct-forming reagents which also
serve as counterions. The extraction of synephrine with a 0.05 M chloroform solution of bis(2-ethylhexyl)phosphoric acid [10] is typical.

Two recent publications describe in some detail the theory and uses
of ion-pair extraction in drug analysis and metabolism studies [11,12].

7. Other Procedures

Problems with recoveries of drugs and metabolites from biological
fluids and tissues have prompted many investigators to develop better

extraction systems. Horning and her colleagues [13] have used salt-solvent pairing to obtain excellent recoveries of drugs and metabolites from urine, plasma, and breast milk. Saturation of the water-diluted biological fluid with ammonium carbonate, followed by extraction with ethyl acetate, resulted in 84% or greater recoveries of various weakly acidic, neutral, and basic drugs. With this method, the amphoteric drug morphine was recovered in 88-100% yield. Excellent recoveries of acidic drugs and metabolites were also obtained, including some glucuronides, by the extraction of urine samples at acidic pH.

Organic extracts of biological materials usually contain large amounts of undesired endogenous materials which can interfere with the analysis of drugs and their metabolites. Immiscible organic solvent mixtures can be used to obtain a partial separation of such impurities from metabolites. If, for example, concentrated extracts from biological fluids are dissolved in small quantities of methanol and the concentrated methanol solution is partitioned between equal quantities of n-hexane and acetonitrile, most of the more polar metabolites and some endogenous materials will partition into the acetonitrile phase, whereas the lipid-like impurities will partition into the hexane phase [14]. This procedure has been used to analyze feces samples. Dog feces extracts were passed down an XAD-2 column, which was then eluted with aqueous methanol. Extraction of the eluate with n-hexane removed lipid-like materials; evaporation of the aqueous phase gave a product which was readily analyzed for the glucuronide conjugates it contained [14].

B. Use of Resins

1. Anion Exchangers

Acidic metabolites can often be extracted from biological fluids by the solvent extraction method. An alternative method which is now being used more extensively is anion exchange. Using this method, excellent recoveries of organic acids from urine have been reported [15-17]. DEAE-Sephadex is the most widely used anion exchanger, but others (e.g., see Refs. 4 and 18) are also suitable. The urine (pH 7-8) is passed down the exchange column followed by water. The organic acids captured on the column are usually eluted with aqueous pyridinium acetate [15-17] or hydrochloric acid [4,19]; the effluent is lyophilized and the residue suitably derivatized for GC analysis. A comparison has been made of methods commonly used to isolate organic acids from urine. This showed that more organic acids and fewer interfering substances were isolated by anion exchange than by solvent extraction [16].

2. Cation Exchangers

Cation exchangers have been used to some extent to isolate basic metabolites from metabolism mixtures. Amphetamine, para-hydroxyamphetamine, and para-hydroxynorephedrine, for example, were removed from a tissue homogenate preparation by adjusting the pH to 6.5 and passing it down a Dowex 50 cation exchange column. Subsequent elution of the column with 4 N ammonium hydroxide eluted the three bases [20].

3. Nonionic Resins

A continued need for a rapid method of screening urine samples for drugs and metabolites has stimulated a search for improved extraction methods. Of the column materials in use, the nonionic resin Amberlite XAD-2 (a synthetic cross-linked polystyrene polymer with a high surface area) appears to have the greatest potential. Extraction methods for biological samples (including urine, blood, serum, bile, gastric contents, and tissues) using XAD-2 resin have been reviewed [21,22]. Efficiency of extraction is dependent on pH, volume, and flow rate of the sample and on the nature and flow rate of the eluant used to recover the adsorbed drugs from the column. Weakly acidic, neutral, and basic drugs (but not acetylsalicylic acid, a stronger organic acid), were efficiently removed to an extent of at least 89% from urine (20 ml) buffered to pH 8.5 ± 0.5 when the flow rate through the XAD-2 column was maintained at 2.5 ml/min and the eluting solvent was acetone or methanol-chloroform [23].

XAD-2 resin removes both conjugated and most nonconjugated metabolites from biological fluids. The metabolites may then be eluted from the resin with methanol. If the eluate is concentrated before being partitioned between larger volumes of chloroform and water, the former solvent will contain nonconjugated metabolites whereas the conjugated metabolites will be found in the latter [24,25].

C. Activated Charcoal

This efficient adsorbent is employed to a limited extent in the removal of drugs of abuse from urine [e.g., 26], but is not used routinely in drug metabolism studies. Perhaps it could be used to more advantage in metabolism studies since it is claimed [26] that most drugs bind completely to small amounts of charcoal (<500 mg/10 ml urine) and are easily eluted from it by small amounts of solvent.

III. SEPARATION PROCEDURES

Many techniques are employed to resolve mixtures of drugs and metabolites into individual components. The vast majority of separations are accomplished using gas chromatography (GC), thin layer chromatography (TLC) and high pressure (or high performance) liquid chromatography (HPLC). Other techniques such as column chromatography (adsorbent, partition, and gel), paper chromatography, countercurrent distribution, and electrophoresis are also encountered. Column chromatography is most often used for initial separations of mixtures prior to the use of more specific separation methods (e.g., GC or TLC).

A. Gas Chromatography

Currently, GC is the most widely used method of separating the components of mixtures of drugs and metabolites. Numerous informative textbooks (e.g., Gudzinowicz [27]) and reviews (e.g., McMartin and Street [28], Riedman [29], Drozd [30], Ahuja [31] on the subject are available. Manufacturers and distributors of GC products (e.g., Analabs, Inc. [32]) also provide information on applications of the method.

GC separations are accomplished on a glass, metal, or Teflon column containing a nonvolatile liquid (the stationary phase), usually coated onto an inert solid support material with a large surface area. The components of the mixture are carried through the heated or occasionally cooled column by an inert carrier gas. They separate from one another according to their partition coefficients between the carrier gas and the stationary phase. When a component elutes from the column, it is detected and displayed as a peak on a recorder. The retention time of the peak (i.e., the time interval between the point of injection and the apex of the recorded peak) is characteristic of—but not unique to—the component giving rise to it, under the GC conditions employed. A peak may also be characterized by its relative retention time. The retention time of a reference compound is determined, and that compound is assigned a relative retention time of 1.00. The relative retention times of all other compounds are obtained by dividing the retention time of each with that of the reference compound. GC data from different sources are more readily compared if relative retention times are quoted.

1. GC Columns

GC columns made of glass, stainless steel, copper, aluminum, or Teflon are available commercially. Drug metabolism investigators usually employ glass columns since they are more inert than columns made of metal and can be used at much higher temperatures than Teflon columns. Glass-lined metal columns are also available. They are more robust than all-glass columns but equally inert. Failure by researchers until 1971 [3,33] to identify hydroxylamines as metabolites of primary and secondary medicinal amines, for example, was due at least in part to catalyzed degradations of these metabolites on heated metal columns or metal attachments to glass columns.

For conventional GC analysis, packed columns are employed. These are typically 1-2 m in length by 2-4 mm internal diameter and are packed with an inert solid support, on which is coated the stationary phase.

Capillary columns, however, are becoming increasingly popular. They are made of glass or stainless steel and are generally 15-200 m in length and 0.25-4.5 mm in internal diameter. With capillary (open tubular) columns, the stationary phase takes the form of a thin coating on the etched or porous column wall. This ensures an adequate carrier gas flow rate. Solid supports are not widely used, although micropacked capillary columns are available. The major attraction of the capillary column is that much better resolution of components of a mixture is achieved compared to what is possible on the more conventional 2 m × 2 mm GC column. For example, the identification of 38 of the many constituents of some <u>Cannabis</u> samples was achieved [34] using a capillary column in a temperature-programmed GC linked to a mass spectrometer.

Chromatographic separations can be performed isothermally (constant column temperature) or by temperature programming in which the column temperature is increased at a preset rate during the analysis with, if desired, preprogrammed isothermal periods before and after the temperature increase. The latter procedure permits a greatly increased analysis speed when solutions containing a wide range of compounds are analyzed.

2. Stationary Phases and Solid Support Materials

There are literally hundreds of stationary phases (liquid phases) used in GC [32,35] and various inert solid supports are encountered [e.g., 32]. The amount of stationary phase used to coat the solid support can vary from what approximates to a monomolecular layer to as much as 30% w/w. Thus the number of different possible prepared columns is virtually unlimited. In practice, however, a small number of stationary phases are used in the majority of instances. Those most commonly employed in drug metabolism studies or gaining in popularity have been identified by Moffat [36] (see Table 1). In the authors' laboratory, the most often used stationary phases are OV-17, OV-101, SE-30, Carbowax 20M, Apiezon L, and Apiezon L + KOH. Undoubtedly, each investigator will continue to have his favorite column materials and the number of commercially available materials will remain high. This is disadvantageous if results from one laboratory are to be compared with those from another. There may be some merit in compiling a short list of "preferred stationary phases" for use in drug metabolism studies, as has been done by analysts involved in screening extracts of biological materials for the presence of drugs [38].

There are relatively few commonly used support materials for GC stationary phases. In drug metabolism studies, the ones most often encountered are identified by Riedman [29] as Chromosorb G, Chromosorb W, Gas Chrom Q, and Haloport F. To this list, Chromosorb 750 should probably be added. The most popular gas chromatographic supports are prepared from diatomaceous earth (kieselguhr), which is very porous and has a high surface area. Supports differ in their densities and hence in the amount of stationary phase that can be applied. Chromosorb W, for example, is a low density support which can be loaded with up to 30% of stationary phase; Chromosorb G has a high density with a maximum liquid phase loading

TABLE 1
GC Stationary Phases Commonly Used in Drug Metabolism Studies

Stationary phase	McReynolds constant[a]	Maximum operating temperature (°C)
Apiezon L	143	300
SE-30	217	300
OV-17	884	300
QF-1	1500	250
XE-60	1785	250
Cyclohexane dimethanol succinate	2017	230
Carbowax 20M	2308	230
SP-2300[b]	2408	250
Diethylene glycol succinate	3555	190
Silar 10C[b]	3682	250
OV-275[b]	4219	250

[a]A measure of the polarity of the stationary phase; polarity increases in direct proportion to the value of the constant [37].
[b]Recently introduced polar phases.

capacity of 5% and is recommended for very polar samples; Chromosorb 750 is a relatively new support material which has a density midway between Chromosorbs W and G—the particles are hard and generate virtually no undesirable fines during coating or packing. It is claimed that only minimal adsorption of polar compounds and minimal decomposition of sensitive compounds occur with this support.

Glass beads are also used as GC supports because of their inertness and their ability to be coated with low loadings of the stationary phase. Commercially available glass beads are of a uniform size and are acid-etched to roughen the surface. This permits the application of a uniform film of the stationary phase and eliminates peak tailing.

Support materials, including glass beads and capillary columns, must be treated prior to coating with the liquid phase (and sometimes after coating) if severe tailing of GC peaks, especially of polar compounds, is to be avoided. Peak tailing when kieselguhr supports are used is triggered by adsorptive and catalytic centers on the supports; this occurs because of the presence on the surface of trace quantities of metal oxides as well as of silanol groups (—SiOH) capable of hydrogen bonding with polar compounds. Mineral impurities are removed by washing with hydrochloric acid, and surface silanol groups are inactivated by derivatization with a silanizing agent such as dimethyldichlorosilane (DMCS):

$$\begin{array}{l} -SiOH \\ -SiOH \end{array} + Cl_2Si(CH_3)_2 \longrightarrow \begin{array}{l} -SiO \\ -SiO \end{array}\!\!\!> Si(CH_3)_2 + 2HCl$$

3. Detectors

There are many techniques by which compounds eluting from a gas chromatograph may be detected, but only five are used to any extent in drug metabolism. One of these, the use of the mass spectrometer as a sophisticated detector, is discussed later. The flame ionization (FI) detector and the thermal conductivity (TC) detector, are in widespread use. They are nonselective, that is, the signal produced by them is approximately proportional only to the quantity of organic material eluting from the GC column. Conversely, the electron-capture (EC) detector and the nitrogen–phosphorus (NP) detector are selective. The response generated by them is dependent on both the chemical nature and the quantity of the material being chromatographed. For this reason, the EC and NP detectors have fewer applications in drug metabolism than the FI detector.

a. Thermal conductivity detector: The TC detector is one of the oldest designs and is still widely used because of its durability, ease of operation, and ability to detect a wide range of organic compounds (lack of selectivity).

The TC detector is not often used in drug metabolism studies because of its poor sensitivity compared to the FI detector. The minimum detectable amount for a TC detector is around 1 μg, which is about 100 to 1000 times less sensitive than the FI detector. TC detectors give a linear response over a wide range of sample amounts (ca. 10^5); this range, however, is somewhat less than that of most flame ionization detectors.

b. Flame ionization detector: Flame ionization detection is the method most widely used in drug metabolism studies. In principle, the effluent from the GC column, mixed with an equal volume of hydrogen, is passed through a metal jet and burned in an atmosphere of air. Combustion of the components which elute from the GC column produces positive and negative ions, and one of these species is collected on a polarized "collector" (sometimes called castle or chimney), situated immediately above the jet. The resulting current is amplified by an electrometer and displayed as a function of time on a recorder. All compounds which combust with ionization in the hydrogen/air flame will give a response in an FI detector. Compounds notably not detected are water, ammonia, carbon disulfide, carbon dioxide, other simple gases, and inert gases. Detector response

sensitivities of compounds of the same molecular weight but different elemental composition vary more with the FI than the TC detector. The response of the FI detector to an organic compound is approximately proportional to the number of carbon atoms it contains and is linear over a slightly
wider range (ca. 10^5 to 10^7) than TC detectors. Sample quantities down to
about 1 ng can be detected. FI detectors require three gas supplies, the
optimal relative flow rates of which are quite critical to obtain maximum
sensitivity and stable detector operation.

c. Electron-capture detector: Due to their selective nature, EC detectors are used much less in drug metabolism studies than FI detectors.
However, their selectivity together with their greater sensitivity make them
ideal in some instances, since they can detect as little as 1 pg of an organic
compound under certain conditions. Electron capture detectors usually
contain a ^{63}Ni or ^3H source which emits relatively high-energy β-particles
that collide with carrier gas molecules (normally 95% argon/5% methane)
to produce a large number of low-energy secondary electrons. When a potential is established in the detector, a small current called the "standing
current" is produced. Sample molecules eluting from the GC column absorb
some of these electrons and reduce the magnitude of the standing current;
the current returns to its original level when the sample has left the detector. This change in current is amplified and inverted to give a positive
peak on the recorder.

The sensitivity of the detector varies enormously depending on the
ability of the eluting compound to absorb electrons. For example, the response of chlorobenzene is 1200 relative to benzene (=1); bromobenzene is
7500; 1-iodobutane, 1.5×10^6; chloroform, 1×10^6; and 2,3-butanedione,
0.8×10^6. The suitability of the EC detector for the analysis of drug metabolites depends on whether they contain one or several halogens or other
functions that might easily absorb electrons, or whether they are amenable
to simple derivatization with halogen-containing reagents such as trifluoro-
acetic anhydride or heptafluorobutyric anhydride. Derivatization with these
reagents gives volatile products which are particularly well suited for analysis by gas chromatographs incorporating EC detectors.

d. Nitrogen-phosphorus detector: N-P detectors are extremely sensitive towards most nitrogen- or phosphorus-containing organic compounds.
They have been available for some time but, because of their instability,
have not until recently been widely used to detect drugs and metabolites.
Greatly improved NP detectors are now available, and use of them for the
detection of drugs and metabolites in urine and other biological fluids is
rapidly increasing.

In some respects, the NP detector is similar in design to the FI detector. The effluent from the GC column is mixed with a much smaller
volume (about one-tenth) of hydrogen, and the gas mixture is passed into
the detector chamber and heated electrically in the presence of an alkali

source (usually a rubidium salt) to form a low-temperature plasma rather than a discrete flame. By a mechanism not yet fully understood, this treatment produces a minute electric current which is amplified and recorded. Low picogram quantities of N- and P-containing compounds are easily detected. The detector is 20,000-40,000 times more sensitive towards nitrogen and 40,000-80,000 times more sensitive towards phosphorus than it is to carbon.

In drug metabolism, the NP detector is particularly useful if mixtures of nitrogenous drugs and metabolites which retain a nitrogen atom are being monitored. Heterocyclic drugs would be particularly suitable substrates since they are unlikely to lose the heteroatom during metabolic reactions. In contrast, acyclic nitrogenous drugs are substantially deaminated when metabolized. Employment of an NP detector to analyze the metabolites formed from such substrates would be unwise since nonnitrogenous metabolites would remain undetected.

4. Derivative Formation

Most drug metabolites are much more polar than the drug from which they were derived and have considerably reduced volatility. Polar metabolites often have long GC retention times and produce asymmetric, tailing peaks. They may undergo "on-column" degradation; sometimes they fail to elute from the column. Such metabolites may be analyzed by GC methods, however, provided they are converted into stable, more volatile derivatives. It is essential, especially if quantitative data are required, that the derivatization method chosen results in the complete conversion of the metabolite to a volatile derivative which is chemically and thermally stable. The choice of the best derivatization reagent depends on the structure of the polar compound. In their review, Crippen and Smith [39] have constructed a detailed list of derivatives of organic compounds suitable for GC analysis. They identified numerous functional groups which require derivatization and suggested what would be the most appropriate derivative. In a more recent review on this subject, Ahuja [31] has identified eight derivatization procedures: on-column reactions, reactions with dialkyl acetals, silylation, esterification, acylation, hydrazone formation, ion-pair formation, and derivatization for EC detection. Methodologies, advantages, limitations, and hazards of each procedure are described and numerous applications listed. Earlier, Riedmann [29] identified silylation, alkylation, and acylation as the most common derivative-forming reactions but also recognized the value in many cases of special derivatives and of on-column pyrolysis.

a. Silylation: This is the most common method of derivatizing polar metabolites. Silylation is the substitution of a trialkylsilyl [usually trimethylsilyl (TMS): $Si(CH_3)_3$] group for the active hydrogen atom of various compounds which possess OH, SH, and NH groups—including alcohols, phenols, acids, steroids and carbohydrates and their thio counterparts, amines, amino acids, amides, imines, and related compounds. TMS derivatives are not difficult to prepare, provided anhydrous reaction conditions are employed. They are safe to handle, and most of them have excellent chromatographic properties [40,41] although isomerization and other undesirable reactions occur occasionally [31]. The various reagents used in silylation reactions, their thermal stabilities, and those of the TMS derivatives have been described; suggestions on reaction solvents, on suitable GC stationary phases, and on GC column conditioning have been compiled [41]. Behavior of TMS derivatives under electron impact is often predictable, and diagnostic mass spectra are usually obtained [40].

An interesting example of the application of derivatization in metabolism studies concerns attempts to identify various keto acids and related compounds [42]. Derivatization of α-keto acids by various methods including silylation resulted in multiple peaks when the derivatives were examined by GC. To avoid these difficulties, various investigators have used oxime formation, usually by reaction with hydroxylamine [43] or methoxylamine [44], followed by trimethylsilylation. The products obtained (Scheme 1) gave single GC peaks, and the identity of each derivative was confirmed by mass spectrometry.

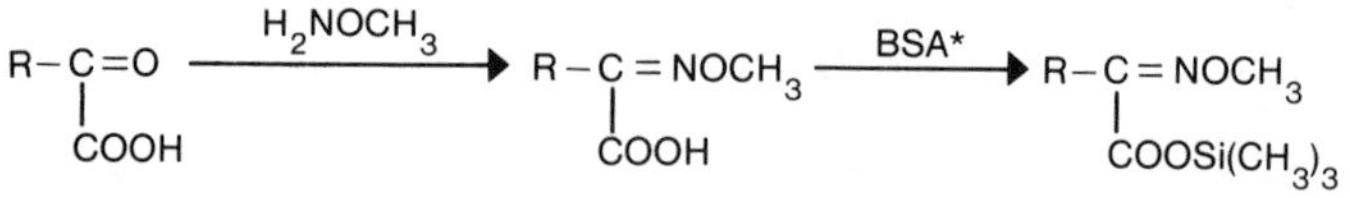

$$R-\underset{\underset{COOH}{|}}{C}=O \xrightarrow{H_2NOCH_3} R-\underset{\underset{COOH}{|}}{C}=NOCH_3 \xrightarrow{BSA^*} R-\underset{\underset{COOSi(CH_3)_3}{|}}{C}=NOCH_3$$

*N,O-Bis(Trimethylsilyl)acetamide

SCHEME 1

b. Alkylation: Acidic drugs and metabolites are generally polar compounds and must be derivatized prior to GC analysis. Diazomethane (CH_2N_2) has been used by many to convert organic acids to methyl esters and phenolic metabolites to methyl ethers, but there are disadvantages to its use—the major one being that many reactive impurities are also methylated and interfere with GC analysis [45].

Esterification of organic acids is readily accomplished by treating the acid with boron trifluoride etherate and an alcohol [46]. The conditions required are very mild, and the presence of other functional groups in the molecule does not interfere with the reaction.

Another versatile group of reagents which can be used to alkylate various metabolites are the dimethylformamide (DMF) dialkylacetals [47]. They possess the general structure I; the reagents which are commercially available have $R=CH_3$, CH_2CH_3, $(CH_2)_2CH_3$, $(CH_2)_3CH_3$, and CD_3. DMF-dialkyl acetals readily react with acids [Scheme 2(a)], alcohols, phenols, primary amines [Scheme 2(b)], secondary amines, and other compounds

a) $R^1COOH + (CH_3)_2NCH(OR)_2 \longrightarrow R^1COOR + ROH + (CH_3)_2NCHO$

b) $ArNH_2 + (CH_3)_2NCH(OR)_2 \longrightarrow ArN{=}CHN(CH_3)_2 + 2\ ROH$

I

SCHEME 2

Quaternary hydroxides in polar solvents form salts with organic acids that react with primary alkyl iodides and produce esters of the organic acid (Scheme 3). Various quaternary hydroxides have been used in this reaction;

$$R^1COOH + Ph\overset{+}{N}(CH_3)_3OH^- \longrightarrow R^1COO^- Ph\overset{+}{N}(CH_3)_3 + H_2O$$

$$R^1COO^- Ph\overset{+}{N}(CH_3)_3 \xrightarrow{R^2I} R^1COOR^2$$

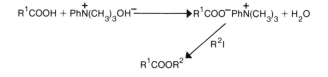

SCHEME 3

one of the best is phenyltrimethylammonium hydroxide [48]. Numerous alkyl groups (R^2) can be introduced by this method. Fluorinated derivatives of acids, phenols (Scheme 4), and sulfonamides, which are ideal for electron-capture GC detection, can be prepared quantitatively by a similar procedure [49].

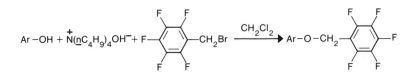

SCHEME 4

Quaternary ammonium hydroxides including tetramethyl-, tetraethyl-, and phenyltrimethyl-ammonium hydroxides form on-column alkyl derivatives of acids, phenols, barbiturates, and other compounds when an extract of the metabolism mixture and the reagent are injected simultaneously onto the GC column. A high injection port temperature is required to complete the reaction [29].

c. Perfluoroacylation: It is now possible to detect and quantitate picogram or smaller quantities of amines and related products by converting
them to suitable fluorinated derivatives. Ahuja [31] identifies the common
derivatives as trifluoroacetyl-, heptafluorobutyryl-, pentafluoropropionyl-,
and perfluorobenzylamines. If an EC detector is used to detect the derivatized
amine, the sensitivity and selectivity of the analyses are greatly enhanced
over other methods of detection. The electron-capture sensitivity of N-(pen-
tafluorobenzoyl)amphetamine is exceptionally high [31], enabling picogram
quantities of this base to be easily determined.

5. Applications of GC to Drug Metabolism Studies

Examples of the routine use of GC in drug metabolism studies are
easily found. Numerous research publications contain original reports and
review articles on the subject. Some journals (e.g., Journal of Chromatography and Journal of Chromatographic Science) are particularly good
sources of information, but many other periodicals and monographs, including those identified in the bibliography at the end of this chapter, contain
excellent examples of the technique. Manufacturers and suppliers of GC
equipment can also provide relevant literature.

One application of GC in drug metabolism studies which is worthy of
emphasis is its use in determining which stereoisomers are formed when
the metabolic process is one which produces a center of asymmetry in the
metabolite [1]. Testa and Beckett [49a], for example, were able to calculate the relative amounts of the (+)-threo, (-)-threo, (+)-erythro, and (-)-
erythro stereoisomers of the amino-alcohol (III) which was formed when
diethylpropion (II) was metabolized in vivo in man. The metabolic products
were derivatized with N-trifluoroacetyl-L-propyl chloride [49b] prior to GC
analysis.

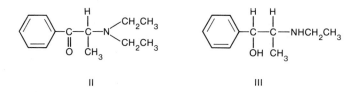

II   III

B. High Pressure Liquid Chromatography

The need for analytical methods of increased sensitivity and stability in
drug metabolism studies has coincided with the introduction of high pressure
liquid chromatography (HPLC; also referred to as high performance or high
speed liquid chromatography) as a routine method of separating and quanti-
tating drugs and metabolites. The technique has wide application in metabolism studies. Three particular advantages of HPLC are that water-soluble

compounds can be analyzed without prior extraction; it is performed at room temperature, which permits the analysis of thermally labile metabolites; it is nondestructive. A disadvantage of the use of HPLC in drug metabolism studies is that it does not directly allow the identification of metabolites of unknown structures.

As in thin layer chromatography, HPLC separations of solute molecules depend on the distribution of these molecules between a stationary and a liquid mobile phase. The relative affinities of solutes for either phase determine solute separation characteristics. Affinity for the stationary and mobile phases may involve adsorption, partition, ion exchange, or a solvation mechanism. The stationary phase is contained within a short, small-bore column through which the liquid mobile phase is forced at high pressure. An efficient pumping system is required to draw the mobile phase from storage reservoirs and to maintain flow rates at constant pressures.

Instrumental and theoretical aspects of HPLC are well documented [50,51] and do not require further elaboration.

1. HPLC columns

Since they have to withstand high pressures (up to 350 atm) HPLC columns are generally made of stainless steel, although some glass columns are available. They are commonly 25-100 cm in length, occasionally much longer, and up to 8 mm in internal diameter. Columns of shorter length (e.g., 30 mm) are gaining in popularity.

2. Column Packings

Several different forms and different particle sizes are available. Adsorbent packings are totally porous and consist of particles in the 5-10 μm range. Because of the small particle size, they offer high capacity and high resolution. Silica is the most commonly used adsorbent; alumina is also used. Adsorbent packings are useful for the separation of numerous classes of organic compounds. Pellicular packing materials are spheroidal in shape and 30-44 μm in diameter. They can be tightly packed in the column and are recommended for the rapid analysis of small quantities of drugs and metabolites.

Polar bonded phase packings for partition HPLC are prepared by chemically bonding a suitable organic moiety such as an oxynitrile group (OCH_2CH_2CN) to a spheroidal solid core material through a Si-C bond. This column packing is useful for the separation of various organic compounds, including polar compounds. Reverse phase packings can be made by chemically combining organic hydrocarbon residues (e.g., octadecyl groups) through a Si-C bond onto a specially prepared silica solid core. This column packing material is most useful for the separation of relatively nonpolar, nonionic compounds including aliphatic and aromatic hydrocarbons, steroids, pesticides, and halogenated compounds.

Anion-exchange HPLC packing materials are produced by chemically bonding a suitable ion exchange group (e.g., quaternary ammonium) through a Si-C bond onto a spheroidal solid support. Cation-exchange packing materials are similarly prepared by bonding sulfonic acid residues onto the solid support. Ion-exchange HPLC is of particular value in the separation of ionic and other polar materials in biological fluids. This application, with an emphasis on the separation of urinary components, has been reviewed by Scott [52].

3. Detectors

After resolution on an appropriate column, the separated components of a mixture are pumped through a detection system. Fixed (254nm) or variable ultraviolet wavelength detectors and refractive index detectors are commonly used; fluorescence and electrochemical detectors are also occasionally used.

4. Ion-Suppression and Paired-Ion HPLC

Extraction of ionic compounds from aqueous biological media (urine, blood, etc.) can be time-consuming and is often incomplete. In addition, mixtures of ionic compounds are not usually separated satisfactorily using conventional gas chromatography or adsorbent or partition HPLC. These facts promoted a search for improved HPLC methods of separating and analyzing the large numbers of ionic body fluid components. High pressure ion exchange chromatography was the initial result; ion-suppression and paired-ion HPLC are alternative techniques.

Ion-suppression HPLC is applicable to the separation of mixtures of organic acids ($pK_a > 2$) and mixtures of organic bases ($pK_a < 8$). It is commonly performed on reverse-phase columns, which operate best with a mobile phase in the pH 2-8 range. A mobile phase buffered to about pH 3.5 ensures that weak organic acids are in their nonionic form (RCOOH) and therefore lipophilic. Similarly, if the mobile phase is buffered to about pH 7.5, weak bases will be nonionized (lipophilic) and will be rapidly separated from a mixture containing other solutes. Strong acids ($pK_a < 2$) and strong bases ($pK_a > 8$), however, remain ionic in the pH 2-8 range and cannot be separated by ion-suppression HPLC.

Paired-ion HPLC permits the separation of strongly ionic compounds by reversed-phase chromatography. A large organic counterion is added to the mobile phase and forms a reversible ion-pair complex with the ionized sample. This complex behaves as an electrically neutral, nonpolar (lipophilic) compound and can be readily chromatographed as a sharp, symmetrical peak on a reverse-phase HPLC column. The lipophilicity of the ion-pair complex formed depends on the sample and on the counterion employed. The more lipophilic is the complex, the greater will be its attraction for the nonpolar stationary phase and the longer will be its retention time. Buffered solutions of counterions are available commercially. Some examples are heptane sulfonic acid and pentane sulfonic acid buffered to pH 3.5, which form ion-pair complexes with organic bases, and tetrabutylammonium phosphate buffered to pH 7.5, which forms ion-pair complexes with organic acids:

$$R-\ddot{N}H_2 + C_7H_{15}SO_2OH \xrightarrow{\text{pH 3.5}} [R+\overset{+}{N}H_3 \ C_7H_{15}SO_2O^-]$$

$$3R-COOH + [(C_4H_9)_4N]_3PO_4 \xrightarrow{\text{pH 7.5}} 3[R-COO^-(C_4H_9)_4\overset{+}{N}]$$

ion-pair complexes

An excellent review of ion-suppression and paired-ion HPLC has been prepared by Waters Associates [53]. A list of 40 drugs which can be chromatographed using paired-ion chromatography is included.

5. Applications of HPLC to Drug Metabolism Studies

Gas chromatography is normally the method of choice for the separation of most drugs and metabolites provided the compounds are lipophilic, capable of being extracted from biological preparations and solutions, and thermally stable (after chemical derivatization, if necessary). When, however, a metabolite is difficult or impossible to extract from aqueous solution (e.g., amphoteric compounds; quaternary amines; glucuronide, sulfate, and other conjugates), is sensitive to pH changes used during extraction procedures, or is thermally labile, then HPLC can be used to advantage.

There are few references to the use of HPLC, as compared to GC, in the drug metabolism literature. In his review, Skillern [54] suggests that the technique is particularly suitable for the quantitative analysis of conjugates of drugs and metabolites, but he admits that there is a paucity of work in this area. He describes the use of HPLC techniques to resolve and quantitate metabolites of acetaminophen, adriamycin, carbimazole, chlordiazepoxide, and indomethacin. A review of HPLC by Tomlinson [55] includes its applicability to the quantitation of drugs with brief comments on metabolites. Clinical applications of HPLC have also been reviewed [56]. Examples are the separation of salicylic acid and its metabolites in a urine sample using paired-ion HPLC (Fig. 1), the analysis of methimazole and its metabolite 3-methyl-2-thiohydantoin in plasma samples from a thyrotoxic patient (Fig. 2), and the analysis of the amphoteric compound para-aminobenzoic acid by paired-ion HPLC using two different counterions [57]. The number of references in the literature to the use of HPLC in drug metabolism studies is slowly increasing. It could be used to greater advantage in the quantitative analysis of amphoteric metabolites and quaternary amines. When instruments which couple high pressure liquid chromatographs to

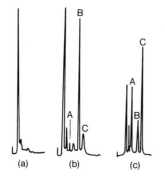

FIGURE 1   Salicylates in urine: (a) urine blank; (b) therapeutic dose;
(c) toxic dose. In the therapeutic range the primary metabolite is salicyluric acid, but in the toxic range this pathway is overloaded and the primary
metabolite is salicylic acid. Peaks: (A) gentisic acid; (B) salicyluric acid;
(C) salicylic acid; column, μBondapak C_{18}, 4 mm × 30 cm; solvent, 30%
MeOH/H_2O and PIC Reagent A; detector, ultraviolet at 313 nm. (From
Ref. 57; reproduced with permission of the copyright owner.)

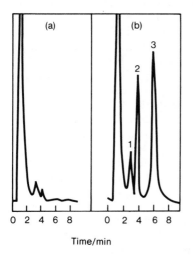

FIGURE 2   Chromatograms of plasma samples from a thyrotoxic patient
receiving methimazole (10 mg) intravenously: (a) control extract; (b) test
extract. Column (10 × 0.46 cm) dry packed with Spherisorb alumina, 10
μm. Mobile phase, 2% v/v methanol in chloroform; flow velocity, 0.17 cm
sec^{-1}; detection, ultraviolet photometer, 254 nm. Peaks: (1) 3-methyl-2-
thiohydantoin; (2) methimazole; and (3) benzamide (internal standard).
(From Ref. 54; reproduced with permission of the copyright owner.)

mass spectrometers become more common, the potential of the technique in drug metabolism studies will be rapidly realized.

C. Thin Layer Chromatography

TLC is employed for various purposes in drug metabolism studies. It is used for the separation and purification of metabolites prior to their characterization by other analytical methods such as ultraviolet (UV), infrared (IR), and nuclear magnetic resonance (NMR) spectroscopy and mass spectrometry (MS). TLC may be used to help identify drugs or their metabolites if authentic reference samples are available for direct comparison of R_f values obtained on two or three different TLC systems. In addition, TLC has been used for the quantitation of compounds which are not amenable to GC analysis, either because of their instability or poor GC properties. The TLC technique can also be of assistance in determining structural features introduced into the drug molecule during the metabolism reaction. A judicious choice of spray reagents (Table 2) can often reveal the chemical nature of the introduced functional group [33, 58-67].

1. Sorbents

Powdered silica gel is the most commonly used sorbent in TLC; alumina, cellulose, and other sorbents are used infrequently. Recent improvements in the quality of sorbents and the consequent improvement in reproducibility of solute separation has made the use of commercially available precoated TLC plates more attractive for metabolism studies. As is true in GC and liquid column chromatography, a narrow and well-defined particle size distribution, a controlled pore size and pore volume, and a specific and graded particle surface area are necessary to minimize spot tailing and maximize solute resolution and sensitivity. Improvements in these factors have led to the development of high performance thin layer chromatographic (HPTLC) plates, designed to be used for the separation of components in the low nanogram or even picogram range—the actual limit being dependent on the nature of the particular solute and the detection system used. Also available are TLC plates which allow reversed-phase chromatographic separation of mixtures of highly polar compounds that would bind strongly to conventional silica or alumina sorbents and not be resolved. The sorbent is manufactured by reacting an appropriate hydrocarbon-silane (e.g., octadecasilane) with the surface hydroxyl groups of a special silica gel. Apart from enabling separations of polar compounds to be made with simple TLC systems, the method is also of value for working out analytical conditions preparatory to reversed-phase HPLC.

2. Solvent Purity

The purity of solvents used both for the TLC system itself and for eluting material from isolated TLC spots is of paramount importance.

TABLE 2
TLC Spray Reagents

Functional group	Reagent	Color	Reference
Nitrogenous bases (amines, hydroxylamines)	Dragendorff	Orange to red	60
Nitrogenous bases (tertiary)	Iodoplatinate	Blue-black	60
Hydroxylamines (or other strongly reducing agents)	Tollen reagent (ammoniacal silver nitrate)	Black (usually without applied heat)	59
Hydroxylamines (or other strongly reducing agents)	Triphenyltetrazolium chloride (TTC)	Pink to red	33, 61
Hydroxylamines	Sodium amminoprusside	Aryl—red to violet; aliphatic—pink or blue	58, 61, 67
Oximes	Cupric chloride	Green	59
Amines (secondary and alicyclic)	Sodium nitroprusside and acetaldehyde	Blue to violet	58
Amino acids	Ninhydrin	Various	59
Phenols	Ferric chloride	Various	59
Phenols	Diazotized sulfanilic acid	Yellow to orange	60
Phenols	Diazotized para-nitroaniline	Red to purple; yellow	60, 62
Phenols	Gibb (2, 6-dichlorobenzo-quinone-4-N-chloroimine	Blue, purple or red	65
Epoxides	Sodium iodide/methyl red	Yellow	63
Dihydrodiols	6N HCl and gentle heat	Yellow	64
Glycine conjugates	Altman (para-dimethyl-aminobenzaldehyde)	Yellow with bright orange fluorescence	65
Glucuronide conjugates	Acid naphthoresorcinol	Red to purple	66

22

Since eluates are often concentrated up to 1000 times (e.g., 10 ml to 10 μl) for GC or MS analyses, trace quantities of impurities in the solvent will also be concentrated by this factor and would interfere in the analyses. All solvents should therefore by purified by distillation or other means before use.

IV. IDENTIFICATION PROCEDURES

Procedures used to identify drug metabolites are varied and depend on whether or not synthetic reference compounds are available for direct comparison of physical properties [e.g., melting point (MP); UV, IR, or NMR spectra; TLC or GC behavior] with those of the metabolite. If the metabolite is of unknown structure, mass spectrometric analysis is almost always necessary to permit at least a tentative identification of the metabolite.

A. Ultraviolet Spectroscopy

UV spectroscopy is usually only of limited use in drug metabolism studies. Most drug and metabolite molecules possess chromophores suitable for UV spectrophotometric analysis, but unequivocal identification of a chemical structure by interpretation of a UV spectrum is rarely possible. If a UV analytical procedure is to be employed, it is essential that all components of a metabolism mixture are completely separated from each other and from interfering endogenous materials extractable from biological fluids. Often complete separation and collection of components is a tedious task, and other methods of quantitative analysis, such as GC or GC/MS, are usually preferred.

    UV spectroscopy can be of value in identifying isolated metabolites, however, if a chromophore is introduced, modified, or abolished by a metabolic process. Hucker and associates [68] made use of UV spectroscopy to help identify two epoxide metabolites of protriptyline (IV) in rat urine. The parent compound gave an absorption maximum near λ 290 nm, which was completely absent in the UV spectra of two metabolites, indicating the olefinic double bond in the 10,11 position of IV was no longer present in the metabolites. Additional data from GC/MS, NMR, and chemical tests enabled identification of the metabolites as 10,11-epoxides of protriptyline and desmethylprotriptyline. The same techniques were also used to identify epoxide metabolites of cyproheptadine [69]. Yamato et al. [70, 71] elucidated the structure of a phenolic metabolite of a psychotropic drug, trazodone (V), partly on the basis of different UV spectra of a basic and an acidic solution of the compound.

Sekine and colleagues [72] used UV spectroscopy to help identify several metabolites of the antibacterial agent piromidic acid (VI). The potential metabolites of piromidic acid were synthesized and spectroscopic data obtained, including their UV spectra. These spectra were classified into three types according to positions of their absorption maxima. The actual metabolites of piromidic acid were then isolated and their UV spectra determined. Comparison of these with the three types of reference spectra provided information on the metabolic fate of the pyrrolidine side chain of VI.

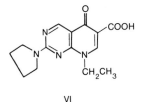

VI

B. Infrared Spectroscopy

IR spectroscopy is rarely, if ever, the method of choice for the identification of drug metabolites; rather, it is used to supplement information gained by techniques such as GC, GC/MS, and NMR spectroscopy. In drug metabolism studies, IR spectroscopy is employed mainly to confirm the identities of metabolites by comparison of their spectra with those of authentic standards. The technique can be useful if insufficient material is available for NMR analysis or where the metabolite is not amenable to analysis by MS. Generally, metabolites are separated by thin layer, column, or gas chromatography and prepared as microdisks (KBr) for IR examination in a spectrophotometer which incorporates a beam condenser. Under these conditions, meaningful IR spectra can be obtained of as little as a few micrograms of a drug or metabolite.

Examples of the value of IR spectroscopy in drug metabolism studies are provided by Douch [73], Porter et al. [74], and Zacchei et al. [75]. Douch [73] separated four metabolites of the fungicide benomyl on a Floricil column and used IR spectroscopy to identify them by comparing their spectra with those of authentic compounds. Porter and associates [74] used IR data to tentatively identify an unusual metabolite of cyproheptadine (VII). The IR spectrum of the isolated metabolite showed bands indicative of C-O and COO$^-$ absorptions and, upon acidification of the sample, a COOH absorption. This, with other data from GC and GC/MS, led to the identification of a

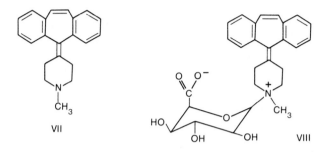

VII

VIII

quaternary ammonium, glucuronide-like conjugate (VIII), as a metabolite
of cyproheptadine in man. Zacchei and colleagues [75] used IR spectrophotometry to identify functional groups in several metabolites of a new
antiarrhythmic drug, MK-251, prior to their complete identification by
means of MS and NMR data. The presence of an absorption band at 1540
cm^{-1}, for example, suggested the presence of a hindered nitro group in
one metabolite. This hypothesis was supported by chemical and accurate
mass data.

C. Nuclear Magnetic Resonance Spectroscopy

Until recently, NMR spectroscopy was rarely used to identify metabolites
in biological fluids because of the insensitivity of the technique compared to
GC/MS and IR spectroscopy. Conventional recording of proton (^{1}H) magnetic resonance spectra requires some 10 to 40 mg of material depending
on the compound being analyzed, its purity, and the information required
from the spectrum. The use of microcells in conjunction with a time-averaging computer (CAT) can reduce the amount of sample required to 0.2-1.0
mg, and the use of Fourier transform NMR spectroscopy (pulse NMR) can
further increase the sensitivity of the system to such an extent that an informative spectrum can be obtained from a 30- to 150-μg sample.

Introductory texts on the theory and applications of ^{1}H- and ^{13}C-NMR
spectroscopy are plentiful [e.g., 76-79], and the uses of NMR spectroscopy
in drug metabolism studies have been reviewed [80]. Utilization of a time-
averaging computer [81] allows repetitive scans to be made of the same
sample. Normally 10 to 200 or more scans are made over a part or all of
the spectrum. The signal due to the compound will always occur at the same
position in the spectrum and thus accumulate faster than the background
noise, which will be random and eventually tend toward a straight line. The
number of scans that may be usefully accumulated usually depends on the
stability of the instrument (in particular, the magnetic field) and the purity
of the sample. Descriptions of the Fourier transform technique are readily
available [e.g., 79,82]. In essence, this technique is also based on the
repetitive accumulation of spectra which result when the sample is repeated-
ly irradiated with an intense radiofrequency pulse. The effect of this

treatment is that all protons in the sample are excited simultaneously, and spectra are therefore more rapidly accumulated using the Fourier transform technique than is possible with CAT-NMR spectroscopy.

Despite the sometimes high sample requirements, the use of conventional NMR spectroscopy to identify drug metabolites is gaining in popularity, in part owing to the availability of less expensive and more sensitive instruments. Routine use of 90- or 100-MHz instruments, for example, is now common. NMR spectroscopy is of particular value if isomeric compounds have to be identified or distinguished. In the following discussion, a few studies which illustrate some applications of NMR spectroscopy in drug metabolism have been selected from the current literature.

Sekine et al. [72] made extensive use of NMR spectroscopy to identify metabolites of the antibacterial agent piromidic acid (VI). Metabolites were extracted from urine, before and after incubation with β-glucuronidase, and purified by preparative TLC. The large initial dose of the drug (1 g per 60-75 kg man) made possible the isolation of four of the eight metabolites as solids in sufficient quantities to allow the recording of NMR spectra as single scans on a 100-MHz spectrometer. Structures were assigned with the aid of spin-decoupling and were subsequently confirmed by comparison of the spectra with those of authentic materials. Unequivocal assignment of the location of a hydroxyl group on the pyrrolidine ring of one metabolite (IX) would otherwise have been difficult.

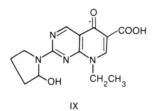

IX

One of the best examples of structure elucidation using various techniques including NMR spectroscopy was reported by Kanai et al. [83], who studied the metabolism of an anti-inflammatory agent, TAI-284 [6-chloro-5-cyclohexylindane-1-carboxylic acid (X)]. Metabolism was achieved in an isolated, perfused rat liver, and metabolites were separated by column chromatography and TLC. Two experiments were performed. In the first,

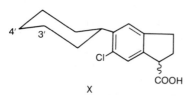

X

the deuterium-labeled drug was used, with a small amount of tritiated drug as a tracer. The isolated metabolites were examined by MS; the main metabolic route was by oxidation at a carbon atom, which was determined to be on the cyclohexyl rather than the chlorindane ring by interpretation of the mass spectra of the deuterated metabolites. In the second experiment, the unlabeled drug, containing only a small amount of tritiated material, was used. Acidic metabolites were esterified and examined by NMR (100-MHz instrument, 17-mg sample size) to determine the positions of hydroxylation on the cyclohexyl ring and their conformations. Proton (^{1}H) assignments were made (a) on the basis of spin-decoupling experiments; (b) after addition of a europium shift reagent [Eu(dpm)$_3$]*; and (c) by comparison of spectra with those obtained from a relevant analog (cis-4-phenylcyclohexanol) of known stereochemistry. In this way, Kanai and associates [83] were able to confirm the identities of 4'-axial, 4'-equatorial, and 3'-equatorial hydroxylated metabolites and further confirm that the last of these metabolites was present as a pair of diastereoisomers.

Hucker et al. [68] have used Fourier transform NMR to confirm that epoxides are formed when protriptyline (IV) is metabolized in different species. NMR signals in the spectrum of IV at $\delta = 7.0$ (vinylic protons, —CH=CH—) were absent from the spectra of two metabolites, having been replaced by signals near $\delta = 4.5$ which were not observed in the spectrum of protriptyline. The investigators concluded that this evidence was in support of epoxide formation. Further evidence was obtained from UV spectroscopy and mass spectrometry experiments and from a qualitative color test specific for epoxides.

NMR spectroscopy has also proved useful in the identification of an epoxide metabolite [69] and a quaternary ammonium glucuronide metabolite [74] of cyproheptadine. Extensive GC and GC/MS data supported these claims.

Kiechel et al. [84] studied the metabolism of the β-adrenergic blocker pindolol (XI). Metabolites were characterized mainly by NMR since they were not amenable to analysis by GC/MS. Two diastereomeric glucuronides of the parent drug were separated by high voltage electrophoresis and identified by comparison of their NMR spectra with that of the parent drug. NMR spectroscopy was also used to identify two isomeric phenolic conjugates of pindolol; the presence of meta aromatic spin-coupling in the

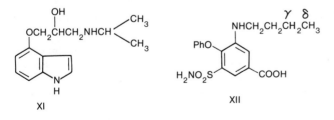

XI   XII

---

*Tris(dipivaloylmethane)europium(III).

spectrum of one metabolite and of ortho coupling in the spectrum of the
other clearly distinguished the isomers.

Kolis et al. [85] used NMR spectroscopy, employing a time-averaging
computer to identify metabolites of the diuretic bumetanide (XII). Metabolic
oxidation of the butylamine side chain gave two isomeric amino-alcohols
which had almost identical mass spectra. Interpretation of the NMR spectra
of the methyl esters of these two metabolites clearly established that they
were γ- and δ-alcohols. In support of this conclusion, the δ-alcohol (secondary) metabolite was found to be optically active, giving a positive rota-
tion when examined by optical rotatory dispersion (ORD), whereas the
δ-alcohol (primary) was devoid of optical activity. An amino-diol metabolite
was also identified by NMR.

Carbon-13 NMR has also been used for metabolism studies, although
the sample requirements of the technique (1-100 mg) are greater than for
proton (^{1}H) NMR. The former technique provides information about the
carbon skeleton and the environment of carbon atoms in the skeleton, which
complements ^{1}H-NMR and MS data.

Examples of the use of ^{13}C NMR in drug metabolism are hard to find,
although studies by Scott et al. [86] provide good instances of its utility.
Metabolism of the anticonvulsant/antiarrhythmic drug mexiletine (XIII) was

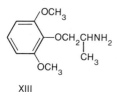

XIII

studied in humans. The major metabolites were isolated as trifluoroacetyl
derivatives by GC and identified by high resolution MS (CI and EI) and by
NMR (^{1}H and ^{13}C). The ^{13}C spectra obtained were particularly clear, and
use was made of both the normal and decoupled spectra for the elucidation
of two ring-hydroxylated metabolites. Subsequent comparison of the spectra
with those of authentic material confirmed their interpretation.

D. Mass Spectrometry

The greatly increased interest in the metabolism of drugs and xenobiotics
in recent years is undoubtedly due to the availability of sensitive and reliable methods of isolating and identifying small quantities of organic compounds. Of all the recent analytically important innovations, the introduction of relatively inexpensive mass spectrometers has been of major significance. Electron impact mass spectrometry (EIMS), chemical ionization
mass spectrometry (CIMS), and—to a much smaller extent—field desorption

mass spectrometry (FDMS) are analytical techniques which are now routinely used in metabolism studies. If an electron impact or chemical ionization mass spectrometer is coupled to a gas chromatograph and a data system, the separation, identification, and quantitation of minute amounts (nanograms or less) of drugs and their metabolites become relatively simple procedures.

1. Electron Impact Mass Spectrometry

When mass spectrometry is employed in drug metabolism studies, in most instances it is EIMS that is used. Molecules are introduced by various methods into the mass spectrometer, where they are vaporized and bombarded with high-energy electrons (0-100 eV). The molecular ion ($M^{\dotplus}$), which is formed initially, has a mass equivalent to the molecular weight of the molecule, and for this reason its presence in a mass spectrum is of extreme importance. Bombardment with high-energy electrons also causes fission of chemical bonds which produces positively charged, negatively charged, and neutral (small molecules and radicals) species. Conventional mass spectrometers measure the mass-to-charge ratio (m/e) and the abundance of each positive ion produced. A mass spectrum is a plot of percentage of relative abundance of each ion produced versus m/e.

The location of the initial positive charge on the molecule generally dictates which bonds will subsequently cleave. Fragmentation, therefore, is not a random process, but rather it results in the reproducible formation of a relatively few number of abundant fragment ions. In addition, ion-ion and ion-molecule interactions occur only rarely and to a very small extent in the mass spectrometer. Thus a compound's mass spectrum is characteristic of that compound and is of considerable value in the qualitative analysis of an unknown drug or metabolite. If the operating conditions in the mass spectrometer are maintained constant, a compound will fragment consistently, yielding ions of the same m/e ratio and in the same relative proportions. Under such conditions, a mass spectrometer is an excellent instrument for the quantitative analysis of subnanogram amounts of organic molecules.

Several distinct types of mass spectrometers are available commercially. All possess sample inlet systems, an ion source (ionization chamber), a mass analyzer (mass filter), an ion detector, and means of displaying and recording the mass spectrum obtained. The major difference in the various types of available instruments is the method by which positive ions are separated in the mass analyzer; most instruments incorporate either magnetic deflection or quadrupole mass analyzers. High resolution instruments utilize magnetic deflection mass analyzers. With such instruments, the masses of all ions in the spectrum are accurately measured to four decimal places or better, which permits an unequivocal identification of the elemental composition of each ion in the spectrum. With magnetic deflection mass spectrometers, however, scan rates are relatively slow.

Quadrupole mass spectrometers are low resolution instruments in which masses of ions are measured to one decimal place. With quadrupole mass spectrometers, however, a rapid scan rate is possible. Typically, up to one scan per second (20-400 amu) can be recorded. A combined GC/quadrupole mass spectrometer/data system is an excellent combination for the analysis of drug metabolites. The effluent from a GC can be scanned every one or two seconds; and by suitable manipulation of the accumulated data, mass spectra of all components of a metabolism mixture, free from spurious background ions, can be obtained. Excellent descriptions of the different types of mass spectrometers and detailed comments on the construction and functions of their component parts are readily available [87-90].

a. Sample inlet systems: Three methods are used to introduce samples into the mass spectrometer. Volatile liquids may be introduced by the HEV (heated expansion volume) method. The sample is allowed to "bleed" first into an evacuated (ca. 1×10^{-1} mmHg) heated reservoir and then in vapor form into the ion source (ca. 2×10^{-7} mmHg or better). This inlet system has very limited use in drug metabolism investigations. Samples can also be introduced into the ion source by means of the direct introduction (or insertion) probe (the DIP inlet). Most solids and high boiling liquids are sufficiently volatile at the very low pressures which exist in the ion source to be analyzed by this method. A sample size of 0.5-5.0 μg generally provides a sufficient number of vaporized molecules to produce a meaningful mass spectrum. The sample may be dissolved in a small volume (1-5 μl) of a pure volatile solvent before inserting it into the tip of the probe. The solvent vapor is rapidly pumped from the mass spectrometer before the sample volatilizes in the ion source.

Generally, samples must be pure if they are to be introduced into the mass spectrometer by the HEV or DIP methods, otherwise a composite spectrum of the compound and the attendant impurities will be obtained. Prior purification of drugs and metabolites is achieved by many techniques, including TLC, HPLC, and column chromatography. Comments on these techniques were provided earlier in this chapter (Sec. III). On occasion it is possible to introduce mixtures of compounds by the DIP method, provided they have significantly different volatilities. If, for example, a mixture of two such compounds is inserted into the mass spectrometer, the initial spectrum will be that of the volatile component and, under ideal conditions, all of this compound will have been volatilized and removed from the instrument before the vapor of the less volatile component reaches the ion source.

The GC inlet system is the method most commonly used to introduce compounds into the mass spectrometer, since only very small amounts of samples are required (ca. 0.01-0.5 μg) and mixtures of compounds can be readily separated prior to mass spectrometric examination. It is important to emphasize that there is an upper as well as a lower limit to the amount of sample that should be introduced. Ion source contamination occurs if excessive amounts are inserted; the detector becomes saturated and its output nonlinear when samples in excess of 1 μg are continuously introduced.

The literature pertaining to the use of combined GC/MS continues to grow at an astonishing rate, such that in the opinion of recent reviewers of the topic [91] it is no longer feasible to write a comprehensive review of the subject. Over 50 books and reviews on combined GC/MS were published between 1973 and 1976 [91], many of which are pertinent to drug metabolism. The review just cited describes practical aspects of, current trends in, and numerous applications of combined GC/MS. Additional comments on applications of GC in drug metabolism studies are described elsewhere in this chapter.

b. Fragmentation: The MS technique may be used to identify drug metabolites without a knowledge of fragmentation processes, provided that authentic reference samples, or a library of reference spectra, are available to permit direct comparisons of spectra. In many instances, however, metabolites are novel compounds, and their structures must be deduced from the manner in which the metabolites fragment in the spectrometer.

Fragmentation reactions depend upon the location(s) in the molecule from where the initial electron is expelled to give the molecular ion(s). If, for example, a molecule contains a heteroatom or π-bonds, fragmentation pathways can often be predicted or explained by localizing the initial charge on the heteroatom (expulsion of an n-electron) or in a region of unsaturation in the molecule (expulsion of a π-electron). A preliminary inspection of the mass spectrum of N-(n-propyl)amphetamine (Fig. 3) illustrates this. The two most abundant fragment ions in the spectrum are the even-electron ions, m/e 91 and 86, which arise as shown in Scheme 5 from the two molecular ions identified as (a) and (b). Molecules containing only σ-bonds, such as the alkanes, produce mass spectra which are least informative since the electron that is expelled to produce $M^{\ddagger}$ cannot be easily predicted. Many alkanes give similar and therefore noncharacteristic mass spectra.

There are many published examples of the use of MS in the elucidation of structures of novel metabolites. Studies on amphetamines have been selected here to illustrate the principles involved. In vivo and in vitro metabolic reactions of various amphetamines in many species have been studied [3,92-94]. N-(n-Propyl)amphetamine [NPA (XIVa)] is extensively metabolized [3,95,96] by various species; five basic, four amphoteric, and three neutral metabolites have been isolated in varying amounts and identified by interpretation of their mass spectra. A knowledge of the mass spectral behavior of the substrate (XIVa) is required in order that the structures of the basic and amphoteric metabolites can be deduced. The origins of all diagnostic ions in the spectrum of NPA (Fig. 3), including those of m/e 91 and 86, are summarized in Scheme 5. If the spectrum of a metabolite of NPA retains the m/e 86 fragment but lacks the m/e 91 ion, it can be concluded that the metabolism site is the benzyl group. In contrast, if the spectrum of the metabolite contains an abundant ion of m/e 91 but no longer possesses an ion of m/e 86, metabolic attack must have been on the $-CH(CH_3)NHCH_2CH_2CH_3$ side chain. By applying these principles, four metabolites of NPA were readily identified as amphetamine (see Fig. 3 and

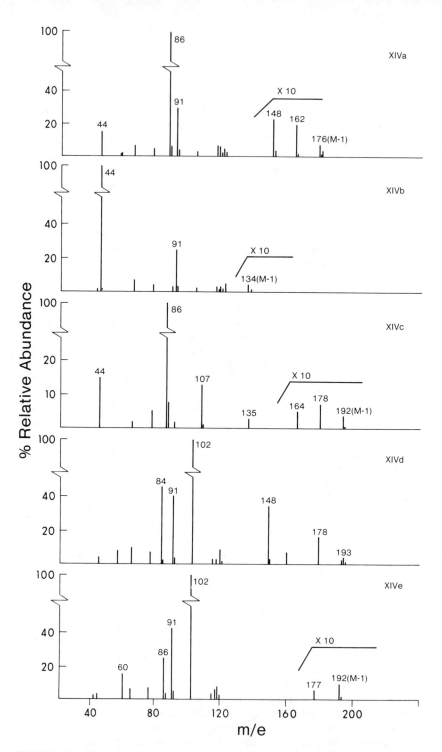

FIGURE 3 Mass spectra of N-(n-propyl)amphetamine (XIVa) and four metabolites—amphetamine (XIVb), 4-hydroxy-N-(n-propyl)amphetamine (XIVc), N-(2-hydroxy-n-propyl)amphetamine (XIVd), and N-hydroxy-N-(n-propyl)-amphetamine (XIVe).

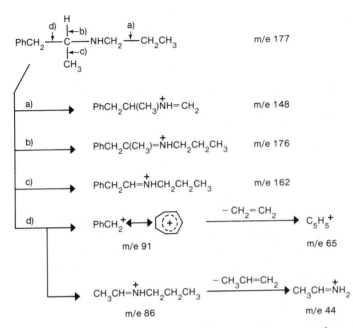

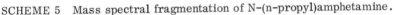

SCHEME 5   Mass spectral fragmentation of N-(n-propyl)amphetamine.

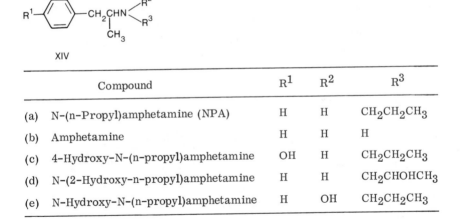

XIV

Compound	R^1	R^2	R^3
(a) N-(n-Propyl)amphetamine (NPA)	H	H	$CH_2CH_2CH_3$
(b) Amphetamine	H	H	H
(c) 4-Hydroxy-N-(n-propyl)amphetamine	OH	H	$CH_2CH_2CH_3$
(d) N-(2-Hydroxy-n-propyl)amphetamine	H	H	$CH_2CHOHCH_3$
(e) N-Hydroxy-N-(n-propyl)amphetamine	H	OH	$CH_2CH_2CH_3$

XIVb); a ring-hydroxylated NPA (Fig. 3) was confirmed by synthesis to be
4-hydroxy-N-(n-propyl)amphetamine (XIVc); and two side-chain hydroxylated
derivatives of NPA (Fig. 3) were confirmed by synthesis to be N-(2-hydroxy-
n-propyl)amphetamine (XIVd) and N-hydroxy-N-(n-propyl)amphetamine
(XIVe), respectively.

Further examples of the use of EIMS in drug metabolism are plentiful in the current literature.

2. Chemical Ionization Mass Spectrometry

One limitation of EIMS is that some compounds do not give spectra containing a molecular ion; the odd-electron molecular ion is often so unstable that it decomposes completely to fragment ions. CIMS is a form of mass spectrometry in which the ionization of the substance under investigation is achieved by reactions in the ion source between gaseous molecules of the substance and reactive ions produced by the ionization of an added reagent gas. Various reagent gases, including methane, isobutane, and ammonia, have been used as a source of reactive ions. Typically, a mixture of methane (>1000 parts) and the sample (1 part) is subjected to electron bombardment in the ion source maintained at a pressure of approximately 1 mmHg. Collisions between electrons and the sample are very few, but the methane is extensively ionized. Various primary ions (e.g., $CH_4^+\cdot$, CH_3^+, CH_2^+, CH^+) are formed which react rapidly with additional methane molecules to give product ions:

$$CH_4^+\cdot + CH_4 \longrightarrow CH_5^+ + \cdot CH_3$$
$$CH_3^+ + CH_4 \longrightarrow C_2H_5^+ + H_2 \quad \text{etc.}$$

The major primary ions produced from methane at >50 eV are $CH_4^+\cdot$ and CH_3^+. The major secondary ions, therefore, have the compositions CH_5^+ and $C_2H_5^+$, and it is these ions which collide with the sample molecule (M) and either donate a proton to the sample, producing an $(M+1)^+$ ion (i.e., MH^+), also termed a quasi-molecular ion (QM^+):

$$CH_5^+ + M \longrightarrow MH^+ + CH_4$$
$$C_2H_5^+ + M \longrightarrow MH^+ + C_2H_4$$

or, abstract a hydride ion, producing an $(M-1)^+$ ion:

$$C_2H_5^+ + M \longrightarrow (M-H)^+ + C_2H_6$$

In addition, ethyl addition ions $(M+29)^+$ are observed with some compounds:

$$C_2H_5^+ + M \longrightarrow (M + C_2H_5)^+$$

All initial ions formed in CIMS are even-electron ions which are not energy rich and have appreciable lifetimes. CI mass spectra are therefore usually much less complex than their EI counterparts. Barbiturates, for example, on electron impact, give rise to molecular ions which are so unstable that they often cannot be detected. In contrast, chemical ionization mass spectrometry with methane provides intense quasi-molecular ions at m/e (M+1)$^+$ for all barbiturates (e.g., see Fig. 4). In this instance, and with many other compounds, no (M-1)$^+$ ion was produced.

Isobutane chemical ionization mass spectrometry is gaining in popularity. When isobutane is the reagent gas, the only significant protonating species that forms is the tertiary butyl ion $(CH_3)_3C^+$, which, compared to CH_5^+, transfers a proton with much less energy—so that at ion chamber temperatures of around 100° mass spectra show a QM$^+$ ion, no (M-1)$^+$ ion, and only few fragment ions of abundances greater than 1% of the QM$^+$ ion. At higher temperatures, more fragmentation usually occurs and spectra are qualitatively similar to that obtained when methane is the reagent gas.

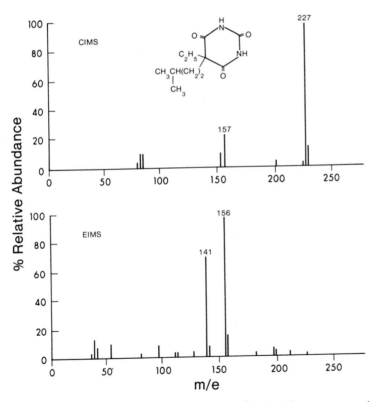

FIGURE 4 Electron impact and chemical ionization mass spectra of amobarbital (molecular weight, 226).

CIMS is generally used to establish the molecular weight of a drug or metabolite. An example is the study by Chang et al. [97] in which the glucuronide of oxazepam was identified by the presence of a QM^+ ion at m/e 823 in the CIMS of the persilylated conjugate (XV); the EI mass spectrum

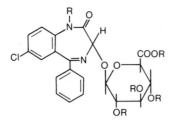

XV,   R = Si(CH$_3$)$_3$

contained no ions of mass greater than 394 amu. CI mass spectra of numerous drugs have been reported [98-100]. In some instances fragmentation does occur, but CI spectra are generally simple and almost all contain abundant QM^+ ions. The base peak in the CI mass spectrum of codeine [m/e (% relative abundance) 301 (4); 300 (QM^+, 18); 299 (5); 298 (7); 284 (4); 283 (21); 282 (100); 281 (6); 257 (3); 255 (3)], for example, is the $(QM-H_2O)^+$ fragment ion shown in Scheme 6. Other metabolism applications of CIMS have been recently reviewed [101, 102].

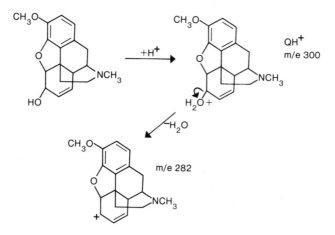

SCHEME 6

3. Field Desorption Mass Spectrometry

FDMS is a relatively new mass spectrometric technique [103,104] by which organic molecules can be analyzed without prior vaporization. The organic solid is deposited on an activated field anode (emitter) which preferably consists of a 10-μm tungsten wire with a dense covering of carbonaceous microneedles, 20-40 μm in thickness. The sample is coated onto the emitter by dipping the field anode into a solution or suspension of the compound. When the field anode is subsequently removed, some of the solution adheres to the carbon microneedles ("whiskers") or remains in the spaces between them. Alternatively, a droplet of the solution can be dispersed onto the field anode from a microsyringe. The solvent evaporates when the emitter is introduced into the FD source.

The field anode is brought to a positive potential of 3-10 kV with respect to ground, and the cathode, a few millimeters distant, to a suitable negative potential so that the potential difference between anode and cathode is about 10-12 kV. Under these conditions, at the tips of the microneedles on the emitter surface, electrons are transferred from adsorbed molecules to the emitter surface by a quantum mechanical tunneling effect [104]. A large fraction of the adsorbed molecules are desorbed in the form of positive ions, which are accelerated and mass-analyzed.

In contrast with other mass spectral techniques, e.g., EIMS, CIMS, and FIMS (field ionization mass spectrometry), in which the sample has to be vaporized before being ionized, the compound suffers less chemical stress in FDMS, which does not require sample vaporization. Thus thermally labile, nonvolatile organic compounds such as sugars and amino acids, can be analyzed by FDMS; no derivatization is necessary. For the production of FD mass spectra of very polar organic solids, the field anode has to be heated. Finding the optimum field anode temperature is very important. At the optimum temperature, the intensity of the molecular ion current is maximal and fragmentation minimal. Several mass scans at different temperatures are usually necessary to determine the optimum field anode temperature.

The detection limit of the FDMS technique is in the neighborhood of 10^{-11} g; it depends on many factors, including the nature of the substance, the solvent and its pH, the morphological structure of the anode microneedles, as well as the sensitivity of the mass spectrometer. The FDMS technique has some major disadvantages. At present it is only suitable for qualitative analysis, although improvements in reproducibility are constantly being made. Other disadvantages are the small, absolute ion current intensities produced and difficulties in establishing the optimum field anode temperature for a compound of unknown composition. In FDMS, an intense peak is often found at one mass unit higher than the molecular weight, sometimes at the expense of the molecular ion. This is due to protonation in the

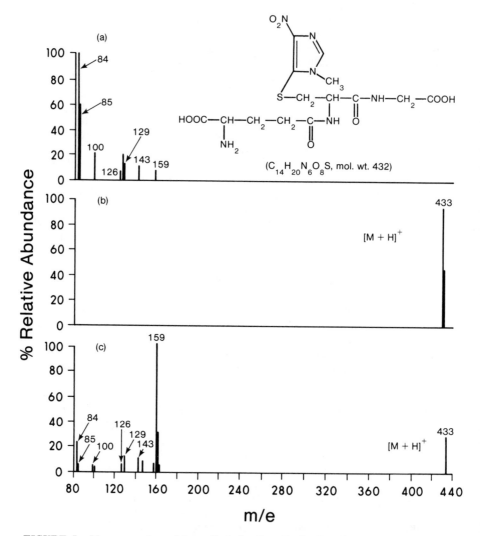

FIGURE 5   Mass spectra of 1-methyl-4-nitro-5-(S-glutathionyl)imidazole:
(a) electron impact, using a direct probe at a temperature of 195°; (b) field
desorption, using 24-mamp emitter heating current; (c) field desorption,
using 27-mamp emitter heating current. (From Ref. 114; reproduced with
permission of the copyright owner.)

adsorbed layer on the field anode. In some instances it is not easy to predict whether the highest mass peak is M^+ or $[M+H]^+$. Criteria which can
be used to make the assignment have been suggested [105]. Other cations,
e.g., Na^+ and K^+, can also be transferred in certain instances to give
$[M+Na]^+$ and $[M+K]^+$ ions.

Recent advances in FDMS have been reviewed [106,107]. Applications
of the technique have also been summarized [104]; spectra have been obtained of pesticides and their decomposition products, glycosides, oligo-
saccharides, amino acids, peptides, nucleosides, nucleotides, drugs, and
drug metabolites including glucuronides. More recent FDMS studies have
been made on mycotoxins [108], pesticides and their metabolic products
[109] and glucuronides [110]. Its use in the area of drug metabolism continues [111,112]. Two examples illustrate the technique. A comparison of
the 70 eV and 18 eV EI mass spectra of neomycin B with its FD mass spectrum was made [113]. In the EI spectra, all ions of significant abundance
were of m/e 205 and smaller and there were no ions of mass greater than
the low abundance ions at m/e 446 and 447. In contrast, 75% of the total
ion current in the FD mass spectrum of underivatized neomycin B is carried
by the $[M+H]^+$ ion (m/e 615). The three fragment ions in the spectrum were
all less than 2% abundant.

Field desorption mass spectrometry was well suited for the determination of molecular weights of azathioprine and its metabolites [114]. In
Figure 5, the EI and FD mass spectra of 1-methyl-4-nitro-5-(S-glutathionyl)-
imidazole are compared. The effect of a change in the field anode temperature is clearly illustrated.

V. QUANTITATION

Accurate quantitation can be the most difficult part of a drug metabolism investigation. Numerous methods can be employed (e.g., TLC, UV spectroscopy, polarography), but only four—radiolabeling, GC, HPLC, and mass
fragmentography—have general application. Quantitation of radiolabeled
metabolites is rarely a specific method of analysis unless combined with
separation techniques such as column chromatography or TLC; further com-
ment on the quantitation of radiolabeled drugs and metabolites is outside the
scope of this chapter.

A. Gas Chromatography and High Pressure
   Liquid Chromatography

The principles of quantitative GC and HPLC are similar. A calibration
curve is first constructed by adding the same quantity of a reference compound (internal standard) to solutions containing different known quantities
of an authentic sample of the drug or metabolite under investigation. The

mixtures are gas-chromatographed and a plot is made of the ratio of the
area (or height) of the drug or metabolite peak to the area (or height) of the
reference compound peak versus the amount of drug or metabolite in solution. When the same quantity of reference compound is added to a solution
containing the drug or metabolite in unknown concentration, and the appropriate ratio of peak areas or heights again determined, the concentration of
the drug or metabolite in the solution can be obtained from the calibration
curve.

The choice of internal standard is important. Since it should have
physical and chemical characteristics similar to those of the compound being quantitated, a homolog or analog of that compound is usually ideal.
2-Methyl-3-ortho-tolyl-4(3H)-quinazolinone (XVIa), for example, was a
suitable internal standard [115] for the quantitation of methaqualone (XVIb).

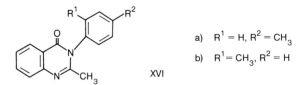

a) R^1 = H, R^2 = CH_3

b) R^1 = CH_3, R^2 = H

XVI

The internal standard should not react with components in the metabolism
mixture. An aromatic ketone would obviously be an unsuitable standard for
the quantitation of hydroxylamine metabolites because of the likely formation of a stable nitrone (XVII).

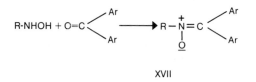

XVII

The accuracy of a quantitative analysis depends on various factors,
some of which were discussed in Sec. III.A on GC and Sec. III.B on HPLC.
Ideally, GC or HPLC peaks used for quantitation should be symmetrical or
virtually so. Asymmetrical peaks are usually due either to overloading of
the column by the compound (the peak tails towards the solvent front) or,
more commonly, to adsorption of the compound on the column (the peak
tails away from the solvent front). Adsorption of a compound on a column
is often difficult to overcome. In the case of GC, silylation of a column will
sometimes mask active sites sufficiently to minimize adsorption. A recently prepared GC column is usually desirable since, with use, stationary
phases gradually bleed from columns, exposing the polar support. In some

cases, the stationary phase itself may be unsuitable for a particular type of compound.

It is desirable for the compound being analyzed and the internal standard to have similar partition coefficients in the extraction system being used. If the partition coefficients are too dissimilar, repeated extractions may be necessary to ensure reproducible quantitative results. Conversely, if the partition coefficients of the drug being analyzed and of the internal standard are virtually identical, as is the case when the internal standard is a ^{2}H- or a ^{13}C-labeled isotope of the compound under investigation, exhaustive extraction of the sample is not necessary. A single extraction might be sufficient to permit accurate quantitation of even poorly extracted drugs.

B. Mass Fragmentography

A major limitation of many analytical techniques is not a lack of sensitivity but rather their inadequate selectivity. Gas chromatography is a selective analytical technique as long as the drugs being analyzed are present in relatively high concentrations (e.g., 1 μg/ml or greater). As the drug concentration becomes lower, the multitude of volatile natural constituents in body fluids or in solvents or materials "bleeding" from the GC column become more prominent in the GC trace and interfere with the analyses. A natural constituent in a urine extract, for example, may have a GC retention time similar to that of a drug or metabolite which is being analyzed. In such an instance, particularly if the compound is present in low concentration, selection of a different GC system is seldom helpful. A way to overcome this problem is to use a more selective detector.

Mass fragmentography, a term introduced by Hammar et al. [116], is a technique which involves the use of the mass spectrometer as a selective detector of components in the effluent from a gas chromatograph. The mass spectrometer is set to detect one or more fragment ions which are characteristic of the compound(s) under investigation. Other compounds present with similar GC retention times but which lack the ion(s) being monitored will not be detected. The method, therefore, combines the resolving power of the gas chromatograph with the specificity of identification and the high sensitivity of the mass spectrometer. Picogram and even lower quantities of metabolites can be detected using the mass fragmentographic technique. Reviews of the technique and its application to drug metabolism studies have been published [102,117-121].

1. Single Ion Monitoring

Most GC/mass spectrometers may be set to record, as a function of time, a trace of the current produced by all positive ions of one particular m/e value. The detection of small amounts of 1-phenyl-2-propanone oxime

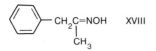

[(XVIII), a metabolite of amphetamine] in rat urine illustrates the single ion monitoring (SIM) technique [122]. When rat urine (50 ml) was passed through an XAD-2 column (1.5 cm × 10 cm), the organic components were retained on the column. They were eluted with methanol and the eluate partitioned between water and chloroform. The total ion GC/MS trace (multiplier gain, 1800 mV) and the SIM (m/e 149) trace (multiplier gain, 3000 mV) of the concentrated chloroform extract are shown (Fig. 6a,b). Another urine sample, to which 50 ng of 1-phenyl-2-propanone oxime (XVIII) had been added, was similarly treated, and GC/MS traces were again recorded in the total ion and SIM (m/e 149) modes (Fig. 6c,d). A comparison of Figures 6b and 6d shows the ability of the SIM mode to selectively detect the oxime in the presence of at least seven other components.

SIM can be used to quantitate very small amounts of metabolites—provided an internal standard is used which elutes separately from the metabolite on the GC. The fragment ion selected for monitoring from the reference compound mass spectrum may differ in mass from that selected for the metabolite. The mass spectrometer can be reset between elution of the compounds to monitor different single ions.

2. Multiple Ion Monitoring

In the multiple ion monitoring mode (MIM; sometimes also called selected ion monitoring*), a mass spectrometer is able to monitor, almost simultaneously, the ion currents due to fragments of four or more different masses (m/e values). This is equivalent to having four or more highly sensitive detectors operating simultaneously. The minimum instrumentation requirements, in addition to a combined GC/MS, are (a) an accelerating voltage alternator (AVA), which changes the accelerating voltage or rf/dc voltage quickly to appropriate values that will selectively focus ions of the required masses onto the detector, and (b) a multichannel recorder. MIM has at least two advantages over SIM: first, two or more compounds may be analyzed simultaneously during a GC/MS run; and second, internal standards may be used which are stable isotope analogs (e.g., ^{13}C or ^{2}H) of the drug being analyzed. The latter advantage can greatly simplify analyses of poorly extracted drugs at low concentrations (low picogram levels), since drugs and metabolites and their ^{13}C- and ^{2}H-labeled counterparts have almost identical GC properties and very similar partition coefficients. Many drugs have been analyzed in urine, blood, saliva, and breast milk using their ^{13}C-labeled analogs as standards, sometimes without prior extraction

---

*The use of the abbreviation SIM can be ambiguous. It can denote single ion monitoring or selected ion monitoring. It is used in the former sense in this text.

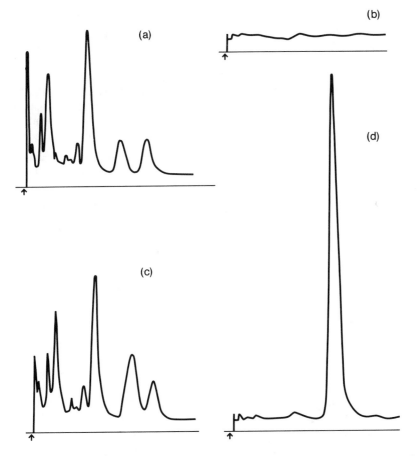

FIGURE 6   GC/MS traces of rat urine extracts. Blank urine: (a) total ion mode; (b) SIM mode (m/e 149). Urine containing oxime XVIII: (c) total ion mode; (d) SIM mode (m/e 149).

[13,123].   Calibration curves are constructed in the same manner as for normal GC or HPLC analyses, namely, plotting the drug to external standard peak area (or height) ratio versus the amount of drug added.

3. Limiting Factors

In many instances, the sensitivity of a mass fragmentographic assay is not limited by the efficiency of the mass spectrometer but by other factors.

a. Internal standards: The proper choice of an internal standard is important. A ^{13}C-labeled analog of the compound being analyzed is preferable since the ^{13}C-atom will not be exchanged or removed during a metabolism study if its position is suitably chosen. However, ^{13}C-labeled compounds are often difficult to synthesize and are expensive if purchased from a commercial source. Conversely, [2]H-labeled compounds are often easy to prepare, but ^{2}H is susceptible to exchange with protons from some solvents. ^{15}N-Labeled drugs and metabolites are also used as internal standards. Excellent analyses may be carried out using internal standards other than a stable isotope-labeled compound, but such analyses are usually less accurate at low concentrations owing to differences in partition coefficient and chromatographic properties of the compound and internal standard.

   b. GC column: Often, the limiting factor in the sensitivity of a mass fragmentographic assay is the efficiency of the GC column employed. In

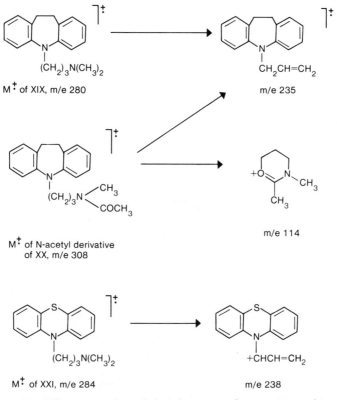

FIGURE 7   Ions selected for the mass fragmentographic analysis of imipramine and desmethylimipramine in plasma. (Drawn from data described in Ref. 124.)

mass spectrometry, low-bleed columns should be used, with stationary phase concentrations of less than 5% w/w of the solid support. However, as the stationary phase concentration is reduced, some of the support may become exposed, causing peak tailing and occasionally decomposition of compounds. Peak tailing is particularly evident at low compound concentrations.

c. Choice of ions: In a mass fragmentographic analysis, appropriate ions in the spectra of the drug, each metabolite, and the internal standard must be selected for monitoring and a calibration curve constructed. Each selected ion should be of reasonable abundance and preferably unique to the particular spectrum—especially if the drug or metabolites and internal standard are not completely separated by GC, as would be the case if a ^{13}C- or a ^{2}H-labeled reference compound were employed. Ions of low mass should be avoided if possible, since they may be common to many compounds. Amphetamine, for example, gives a base peak of m/e 44 which accounts for the majority of the ion current; however, a fragment of m/e 44 also occurs in the spectra of other compounds, including endogenous urine components and some GC column stationary phases.

An example of MIM is provided in the studies by Pantarotto and colleagues [124], who quantitatively analyzed imipramine (XIX) and its major metabolite, desmethylimipramine (XX), in plasma. Promazine (XXI) was used as the internal standard because of its chemical and mass spectral similarity to imipramine, and desmethylimipramine was analyzed as its N-acetyl derivative. The ions selected for the mass fragmentographic study were of m/e 114, 235, 238, 280, 284, and 308 and are identified in Figure 7. Additional applications of mass fragmentography in drug metabolism studies are presented in excellent reviews by Carrington and Frigerio [120] and Pantarotto et al. [124].

VI. CONCLUSION

In addition to a sound understanding of known metabolic transformations and of the chemistry of functional groups, it is of paramount importance in drug metabolism studies to have a good appreciation of the analytical techniques that are used so as to ensure that they are applied properly and that accumulated data are accurately interpreted. The principle methods used for the extraction, separation, identification, and quantitation of drug metabolites, excluding radiochemical techniques, have been described in this chapter.

In studies on the metabolism of drugs, numerous analytical techniques can be employed—although only a few of them are generally used in any one investigation. Many methods of extraction have been described; usually those which are suitable for studies on urine and plasma are also applicable to the extraction of feces and bile samples. Some investigators routinely use resins to remove metabolites from biological samples, whereas others prefer to extract biological samples with organic solvents or use other extraction methods. The choice of the extraction method is often an arbitrary one. Extraction of drugs and metabolites by the ion-pairing technique is probably a greatly underused method.

In earlier metabolism studies, TLC and UV spectroscopy were widely used in the identification of metabolites, especially when authentic samples of the metabolites were available to permit direct comparisons of their TLC and UV properties. The use of these techniques to identify metabolites has declined, having been superseded by more specific methods of analysis. TLC now plays a more important role in the separation of drugs and metabolites prior to the application of other analytical techniques, including NMR and IR spectroscopy, GC, and MS.

The introduction of combined GC/MS has revolutionized drug metabolism studies. The use of capillary column GC combined with MS and of SIM have greatly improved both the selectivity and the sensitivity of the method. A wider use of field desorption and of atmospheric pressure MS will undoubtedly aid future drug metabolism studies.

HPLC is an analytical technique which is finding more application in drug metabolism studies, particularly with those compounds which are not easily examined by GC because they are either thermolabile or too polar. Combined HPLC/mass spectrometers have recently become available commercially. Improvements in their design will lead to an increased use of HPLC in the separation, identification, and quantitation of metabolites.

NMR is used increasingly for the elucidation of drug metabolite structures as a result of the introduction of relatively inexpensive high resolution NMR spectrometers incorporating Fourier transform analysis.

The stereochemical aspects of drug metabolism are receiving increasing attention. Consequently, the resolution and quantitation of optical isomers and diastereoisomers is of great importance. Chiral derivatization reagents are valuable for the separation and quantitation of isomers using GC.

Numerous other analytical techniques, such as polarography and optical rotatory dispersion, are used occasionally in metabolic investigations. In some instances, special analytical techniques are of particular value in characterizing metabolites. Undoubtedly, improvements in analytical techniques will continue to be made and progress in the study of drug metabolism will be sustained.

REFERENCES

1. B. Testa and P. Jenner, in Drug Fate and Metabolism: Methods and Techniques (E. R. Garrett and J. L. Hirtz, eds.), Vol. 2. Dekker, New York, 1978, pp. 143-193.
1a. H. B. Hucker, A. J. Balletto, J. Demetriades, B. H. Arison, and A. G. Zacchei, Drug Metab. Dispos. $\underline{5}$:132 (1977).

2. A. Zltakis and K. Kim, J. Chromatogr. 126:475 (1976).
3. R. T. Coutts and A. H. Beckett, Drug Metab. Rev. 6:51 (1977).
4. C. Lin, Y. Li, J. McGlotten, J. B. Morton, and S. Symchowicz, Drug Metab. Dispos. 5:234 (1977).
5. G. Schill, Acta Pharm. Suec. 2:13 (1965).
6. B.-A. Persson and B. L. Karger, J. Chromatogr. Sci. 12:521 (1974).
7. P. F. G. Boon and A. W. Mace, J. Chromatogr. 41:105 (1969).
8. B. Fransson and G. Schill, Acta Pharm. Suec. 12:107, 417 (1975).
9. T. Nordgren and R. Modin, Acta Pharm. Suec. 12:407 (1975).
10. R. Modin and M. Johansson, Acta Pharm. Suec. 8:561 (1971).
11. G. Schill, K. O. Borg, R. Modin, and B. A. Persson, in Progress in Drug Metabolism (J. W. Bridges and L. F. Chasseaud, eds.), Vol. 2. Wiley, New York, 1977, pp. 219-258.
12. G. Schill, R. Modin, K. O. Borg, and B. A. Persson, in Drug Fate and Metabolism: Methods and Techniques (E. R. Garrett and J. L. Hirtz, eds.), Vol. 1. Dekker, New York, 1977, pp. 135-185.
13. M. G. Horning, P. Gregory, J. Nowlin, M. Stafford, K. Lertratan-angkoon, C. Butler, W. G. Stillwell, and R. M. Hill, Clin. Chem. 20: 282 (1974).
14. Y. Yanagi, F. Haga, M. Endo, and S. Kitagawa, Xenobiotica 6:101 (1976)
15. E. C. Horning and M. G. Horning, Clin. Chem. 17:802 (1971).
16. J. A. Thompson and S. P. Markey, Anal. Chem. 47:1313 (1975).
17. A. M. Lawson, R. A. Chalmers, and R. W. E. Watts, Clin. Chem. 22:1283 (1976).
18. E. Nakamura, L. E. Rosenberg, and K. Tanaka, Clin. Chim. Acta 68:127 (1976).
19. R. H. Horrocks, E. J. Hindle, P. A. Lawson, D. H. Orrell, and A. J. Poole, Clin. Chim. Acta 69:93 (1976).
20. B. B. Brodie, A. K. Cho, and G. L. Gessa, in Amphetamines and Related Compounds (E. Costa and S. Garattini, eds.), Raven Press, New York, 1970, p. 217.
21. A. Stolman and P. A. F. Pranitis, Clin. Toxicol. 10:49 (1977).
22. Technical Bulletin No. 10, Applied Science Laboratories Inc., P.O. Box 440, State College, Pa.
23. M. P. Kullberg and C. W. Gorodetzky, Clin. Chem. 20:177 (1974).
24. A. Karim, J. Hribar, W. Aksamit, M. Doherty, and L. J. Chinn, Drug Metab. Dispos. 3:467 (1975).
25. Y. Kishimoto, S. Kraychy, and R. E. Ranney, Xenobiotica 2:237 (1972).
26. J. M. Meola and M. Vanko, Clin. Chem. 20:184 (1974).
27. B. J. Gudzinowicz, Gas Chromatographic Analysis of Drugs and Pesticides. Dekker, New York, 1967.
28. C. McMartin and H. V. Street, J. Chromatogr. 22:274 (1966).
29. M. Riedmann, Xenobiotica 3:411 (1973).
30. J. Drozd, J. Chromatogr. 113:303 (1975).
31. S. Ahuja, J. Pharm. Sci. 65:163 (1976).

32. Catalog 18 (June 27, 1976), Analabs, Inc., 80 Republic Drive, North Haven, Conn.

33. A. H. Beckett and S. Al-Sarraj, J. Pharm. Pharmacol. 25:328 (1973).

34. M. Novotny, M. L. Lee, C.-E. Low, and A. Raymond, Anal. Chem. 48:24 (1976).

35. S. T. Preston, J. Chromatogr. Sci. 8:18A (1970).

36. A. C. Moffat, Proc. Anal. Div. Chem. Soc. 13:355 (1976).

37. W. O. McReynolds, J. Chromatogr. Sci. 8:685 (1970).

38. A. C. Moffat, J. Chromatogr. 113:69 (1975).

39. R. C. Crippen and C. E. Smith, J. Gas Chromatogr. 3:37 (1965).

40. A. E. Pierce, Silylation of Organic Compounds. Pierce Chemical Co., Rockford, Ill., 1968.

41. Pierce Handbook and General Catalog, 1977-1978. Pierce Chemical Co., Box 117, Rockford, Ill., pp. 214-243.

42. E. Jellum, J. Chromatogr. 143:427 (1977).

43. H. J. Sternowsky, J. Roboz, F. Hutterer, and G. Gaull, Clin. Chim. Acta 47:371 (1973).

44. M. G. Horning, E. A. Boucher, A. M. Moss, and E. C. Horning, Anal. Lett. 1:713 (1968).

45. J. Horner, S. S. Que Hee, and R. G. Sutherland, Anal. Chem. 46: 110 (1974).

46. P. K. Kadaba, J. Pharm. Sci. 63:1333 (1974).

47. See Ref. 41, pp. 253-255.

48. R. H. Greeley, J. Chromatogr. 88:229 (1974).

49. See Ref. 41, pp. 257 and 263.

49a. B. Testa and A. H. Beckett, J. Pharm. Pharmacol. 25:119 (1973).

49b. J. W. Westley and B. Halpern, in Gas Chromatography 1968 (C. L. A. Harbourn, ed.). Inst. of Petroleum, London, 1969, pp. 119-128.

50. N. Hadden, F. Baumann, F. MacDonald, M. Munk, R. Stevenson, D. Gere, F. Zamaroni, and R. Majors, in Basic Liquid Chromatography. Varian Aerograph, Walnut Creek, Calif., 1972.

51. P. M. Rajcsanyi and E. Rajcsanyi, in High-Speed Liquid Chromatography. Dekker, New York, 1975.

52. C. D. Scott, Science 186:226 (1974).

53. Waters Associates, Inc., Paired-Ion Chromatography—An Alternative to Ion-Exchange. Milford, Mass., 1976.

54. G. G. Skellern, Proc. Anal. Div. Chem. Soc. 13:357 (1976).

55. E. Tomlinson, Pharm. J. 220:13 (1978).

56. I. M. House and D. J. Berry, in High Pressure Liquid Chromatography in Clinical Chemistry (P. F. Dixon, C. H. Gray, C. K. Lim, and M. S. Stoll, eds.). Academic Press, New York, 1976, p. 155.

57. Waters Associates, Inc., Analysis of Pharmaceutical Products. Milford, Mass., 1977.

58. F. Feigl, in Spot Tests in Organic Analysis. Elsevier, Amsterdam. 1966.

59. K. G. Krebs, D. Heusser, and H. Wimmer, in Thin-Layer Chromatography: A Laboratory Handbook (E. Stahl, ed.), 2nd ed. Springer, New York, 1969, p. 854.
60. E. G. C. Clark, in Isolation and Identification of Drugs, Vol. 1. Pharmaceutical Press, London, 1969, p. 797.
61. A. H. Beckett and P. M. Belanger, Xenobiotica 4:509 (1974).
62. G. E. R. Hook and J. N. Smith, Biochem. J. 102:504 (1967).
63. F. Oesch, D. M. Jerina, and J. W. Daly, Arch. Biochem. Biophys. 144:253 (1971).
64. J. Rigaudy and L. Nedelec, Bull. Soc. Chim. France, p. 400 (1960).
65. I. Smith, J. W. T. Seakins, and J. Dayman, in Chromatographic and Electrophoretic Techniques (I. Smith, ed.), 3rd ed., Vol. 1. Heinemann, London, 1969, pp. 125 and 371.
66. R. M. C. Dawson, D. C. Elliott, W. H. Elliott, and K. M. Jones (eds.), Data for Biochemical Research. Oxford Univ. Press, London, 1969.
67. A. H. Beckett and S. Al-Sarraj, J. Pharm. Pharmacol. 25:335 (1973).
68. H. B. Hucker, A. J. Balletto, J. Demetriades, B. H. Arison, and A. G. Zacchei, Drug Metab. Dispos. 3:80 (1975).
69. H. B. Hucker, A. J. Balletto, S. C. Stauffer, A. G. Zacchei, and B. H. Arison, Drug Metab. Dispos. 2:406 (1974).
70. C. Yamato, T. Takahashi, and T. Fujita, Xenobiotica 4:313 (1974).
71. C. Yamato, T. Takahashi, T. Fujita, S. Kuriyama, and N. Hirose, Xenobiotica 4:765 (1974).
72. Y. Sekine, M. Miyamoto, M. Hashimoto, and K. Nakamura, Xenobiotica 6:185 (1976).
73. P. G. C. Douch, Xenobiotica 3:367 (1973).
74. C. C. Porter, B. H. Arison, V. F. Gruber, D. C. Titus, and W. J. A. Vandenheuvel, Drug Metab. Dispos. 3:189 (1975).
75. A. G. Zacchei, L. L. Weidner, G. H. Besselaar, and E. B. Raftery, Drug Metab. Dispos. 4:387 (1976).
76. J. R. Dyer, Applications of Absorption Spectroscopy of Organic Compounds. Prentice-Hall, Englewood Cliffs, N.J., 1965.
77. R. H. Bible, Interpretation of NMR Spectra: An Empirical Approach. Plenum Press, New York, 1965.
78. L. M. Jackman and S. Sternhell, Application of Nuclear Magnetic Resonance Spectroscopy in Organic Chemistry. Pergamon Press, Oxford, 1969.
79. G. C. Levy and G. L. Nelson, Carbon-13 Nuclear Magnetic Resonance for Organic Chemists. Wiley (Interscience), New York, 1972.
80. D. E. Case, Xenobiotica 3:451 (1973).
81. L. C. Allen and L. F. Johnson, J. Amer. Chem. Soc. 85:2668 (1963).
82. R. R. Ernst, Advan. Magnetic Resonance 2:1 (1966).
83. Y. Kanai, T. Kobayashi, and S. Tanayama, Xenobiotica 3:657 (1973).
84. J. R. Kiechel, P. Nicklaus, E. Schreier, and H. Wagner, Xenobiotica 5:741 (1975).

85. S. J. Kolis, T. H. Williams, and M. A. Schwartz, Drug Metab. Dispos. 4:169 (1976).

86. K. N. Scott, M. W. Couch, B. J. Wilder, and C. M. Williams, Drug Metab. Dispos. 1:506 (1973).

87. H. C. Hill, Introduction to Mass Spectrometry. Heyden, London, 1966.

88. W. H. McFadden, Techniques of Combined Gas Chromatography/ Mass Spectrometry: Applications in Organic Analysis. Wiley (Interscience), New York, 1973.

89. H. H. Willard, L. L. Merritt, Jr., and J. A. Dean, Instrumental Methods of Analysis, 4th ed. Van Nostrand, New York, 1965, pp. 435-443.

90. J. T. Watson, Introduction to Mass Spectrometry: Biomedical, Environmental and Forensic Applications. Raven Press, New York, 1976.

91. C. J. W. Brooks and B. S. Middleditch, in Mass Spectrometry: A Specialist Periodical Report (R. A. W. Johnstone), sen. reporter), Vol. 4. Chemical Soc., London, 1977, p. 146.

92. E. Costa and S. Garattini (eds.), International Symposium on Amphetamines and Related Compounds. Raven Press, New York, 1970.

93. E. Usdin and S. Snyder (eds.), Frontiers in Catecholamine Research. Pergamon Press, Oxford, 1973.

94. J. Caldwell, Drug Metab. Rev. 5:219 (1976).

95. R. T. Coutts, G. W. Dawson, and A. H. Beckett, J. Pharm. Pharmacol. 28:815 (1976).

96. R. T. Coutts, G. W. Dawson, C. W. Kazakoff, and J. Y. Wong, Drug Metab. Dispos. 4:256 (1976).

97. T. T. L. Chang, C. F. Kuhlman, R. T. Schillings, S. F. Sisenwine, C. O. Tio, and H. W. Ruelius, Experientia 29:653 (1973).

98. H. M. Fales, G. W. A. Milne, and T. Axenrod, Anal. Chem. 42:1432 (1970).

99. G. W. A. Milne, H. M. Fales, and T. Axenrod, Anal. Chem. 43:1815 (1971).

100. R. Saferstein, J.-M. Chao, and J. Manura, J. Forensic Sci. 19:463 (1974).

101. R. T. Parfitt, Pharm. J. 216:109 (1976).

102. B. J. Millard, in Mass Spectrometry: A Specialist Periodic Report (R. A. W. Johnstone, sen. reporter), Vol. 4. Chemical Soc., London, 1977, p. 186.

103. H. D. Beckey, Angew. Chem. Intern. Ed. Engl. 8:623 (1969).

104. H. D. Beckey and H.-R. Schulten, Angew. Chem. Intern. Ed. 14:403 (1975).

105. H.-R. Schulten and H. D. Beckey, Org. Mass Spectrom. 9:1154 (1974).

106. J. M. Wilson, in Mass Spectrometry: A Specialist Periodic Report (R. A. W. Johnstone, sen. reporter), Vol. 4. Chemical Soc., London, 1977, p. 102.

107. P. J. Derrick, in Mass Spectrometry: A Specialist Periodic Report (R. A. W. Johnstone, sen. reporter), Vol. 4. Chemical Soc., London, 1977, p. 132.

108. J. A. Spohn, P. A. Dreifuss, and H.-R. Schulten, J. Ass. Offic. Anal. Chemists 60:73 (1977).

109. H.-R. Schulten, J. Agr. Food Chem. 24:743 (1976).

110. R. T. Parfitt, D. E. Games, M. Rossiten, M. S. Rogers, and A. Weston, Biomed. Mass Spectrom. 3:232 (1976).

111. H.-R. Schulten, Cancer Treat. Repts. 60:501 (1976).

112. D. A. Brent, J. Ass. Offic. Anal. Chemists 59:1006 (1976).

113. K. L. Rinehart, J. C. Cook, K. H. Maurer, and U. Rapp, J. Antibiot. 27:1 (1974).

114. D. A. Brent, P. deMiranda, and H.-R. Schulten, J. Pharm. Sci. 63:1370 (1974).

115. C. N. Reynolds, K. Wilson, and D. Burnett, Xenobiotica 6:113 (1976).

116. C.-G. Hammar, B. Holmstedt, and R. Ryhage, Anal. Biochem. 25:532 (1968).

117. C.-G. Hammar, B. Holmstedt, J.-E. Lindgren, and R. Tham, Advan. Pharmacol. Chemother. 7:53 (1969).

118. A. E. Gordon and A. Frigerio, J. Chromatogr. 73:401 (1972).

119. B. J. Millard, in Progress in Drug Metabolism (J. W. Bridges and L. F. Chasseaud, eds.), Vol. 1. Wiley (Interscience), New York, 1976.

120. R. Carrington and A. Frigerio, Drug Metab. Rev. 6:243 (1977).

121. A. Frigerio and N. Castagnoli (eds.), Mass Spectrometry in Biochemistry and Medicine. Raven Press, New York, 1974.

122. R. T. Coutts and G. R. Jones, unpublished results (1977).

123. M. G. Horning, W. G. Stillwell, J. Nowlin, K. Lertratanangkoon, D. Carroll, I. Dzidic, R. N. Stillwell, and E. C. Horning, J. Chromatogr. 91:413 (1974).

124. C. Pantarotto, G. Belvedere, L. Burti, and A. Frigerio, Advan. Mass Spectrom. Biochem. Med. 1:433 (1976).

Chapter 2

A STRUCTURAL APPROACH TO SELECTIVITY IN DRUG METABOLISM AND DISPOSITION

Bernard Testa

Department of Medicinal Chemistry
School of Pharmacy
University of Lausanne
Lausanne, Switzerland

Peter Jenner

Department of Neurology
Institute of Psychiatry
and
King's College Hospital Medical School
London, England

The metabolism and disposition of a drug substrate is governed by the relationship between the nature of the biological system concerned and the inherent properties of the drug molecule. This implies that distinct but closely related substrates may exhibit a different metabolic behavior (substrate selectivity) or that the same substrate may give rise to two or more metabolites at different rates and by competitive pathways (product selectivity). We have therefore attempted in this chapter to apply concepts of structural chemistry to analyze examples of both substrate and product selectivity in terms of the enzymic discrimination of analogous, homologous, regioisomeric, diastereoisomeric, and enantiomeric substrates, together with regiotopic, diastereotopic, and enantiotopic groups. All of these factors are of importance in determining the overall metabolism of drug molecules, and by this approach we have built up a qualitative view of the nature of enzymic mechanisms and enzyme-substrate interactions. Recent advances in this field have also shown that some form of quantitative assessment of the influence of chemical and physicochemical factors on drug metabolism and disposition can be obtained by the use of QSAR techniques. We have therefore examined the uses and limitations of this approach as presently applied in explaining and predicting the metabolic fate of groups of closely related substrates.

We believe that the extension of this type of study is of notable importance to overall structure-activity relationships and may be broadly useful in the future design of drug molecules and in drug development as a whole.

I. INTRODUCTION

When molecules (endogenous or exogenous) undergo biotransformation, they interact with biological systems (enzymes, enzymic systems, cells, tissues, organs, or organisms) characterized by higher organizational states of matter. As a result, understanding drug metabolism calls for a multidisciplinary approach—an approach which can be schematically considered as involving, on one side, physical sciences (e.g., chemistry, physicochemistry) and, on the other side, life sciences (e.g., enzymology, pharmacology, toxicology). Selectivity* aspects of drug metabolism and disposition constitute the context of this chapter and are ideally discussed within this perspective. From a biological point of view, enzyme selectivity is a corollary of biological recognition. There are two aspects of enzyme selectivity, namely, recognition of the substrate by formation of an enzyme–substrate complex (binding selectivity) and recognition of the transition state by catalysis of the reaction (kinetic selectivity). In either case, however, selectivity

---

*Chemists label as "stereoselective" those reactions in which one stereoisomer is either formed or converted preferentially to the other stereoisomer(s); on the other hand, a "stereospecific" reaction converts stereoisomeric starting materials to contrasting stereoisomeric products [1,2]. In biochemistry, these two aspects of stereoreactivity are often intermingled and as a result, stereoselectivity and stereospecificity are rarely distinguished [2]. Pharmacologists use the terms stereoselectivity and stereospecificity with yet other meanings [3]. To avoid this confusion, the term specificity will not be employed in the present chapter. Rather, use will be made here of the term substrate selectivity to designate a situation where isomeric substrates are consumed at different rates in a given reaction, and product selectivity when a given substrate yields isomeric products in different amounts [4,5]. When isomeric substrates generate isomeric products in contrasting ratios, the term substrate-product selectivity is used [5]. It should be noted that selectivity can be quantified, e.g., low, marked, high, complete, or 90% selectivity.

stems from the structural complementarity of the partners in a complex
[6,7]. The structure of substrates is thus a key factor in the selectivity
phenomenon, and without neglecting enzymic aspects our attention here will
be focused mainly on substrate structure. Viewing drug metabolism through
the eye of a structural chemist increases considerably our understanding of
drug metabolism and our ability to rationalize the flood of data which threatens modern scientists [8].

At this stage, some explanations are necessary as to the meaning of
the word structure. The term usually refers to the three-dimensional
geometry of chemical entities. However, current chemical models can be
envisaged as being multidimensional [9]. Thus, a temporal dimension must
be added if conformational properties are to be considered. Further, one
might like to consider electronic terms as additional dimension(s), and
electronic properties as the parameters occupying these dimensions.

In our mind, the concept of "structure" must have a meaning as general and as far-reaching as possible by encompassing a multidimensional
visualization of molecules. We therefore include in the concept of structure
not only the geometry and steric properties of molecules but also electronic
and derived properties such as ionization and solubilities.

The present contribution considers the various approaches which have
proved of value in assessing the influence of substrate structure on drug
metabolism and disposition. Some of these approaches have already been
reviewed individually and with a systematic presentation of data [e.g., 5,
10-13]. In the pages that follow, only selected and representative studies
will be discussed, the purpose of these examples being to reveal and illustrate the underlying structural concepts.

II. SUBSTRATE SELECTIVITY TOWARD ANALOGS AND
    HOMOLOGS: A QUALITATIVE APPROACH

Studies investigating the fate of a single compound yield results whose va-
lidity is a priori limited to that compound and experimental conditions.
Only upon comparing the results with those for other compounds and conditions can some generalizations be ventured. Similarly, studies involving
small series of homologs or analogs again yield results of relatively limited
value. In particular, generalizing and extrapolating the results to other
derivatives calls for great caution. However, the use of carefully selected
series can lead to fruitful and sound conclusions. The several examples to
be discussed in this chapter have been selected for their interest and diversity in illustrating the above argument.

All studies involving limited series of compounds can only lead to
qualitative correlations between structural properties of substrates and
their fate. Correlations of a quantitative nature require larger sets of
molecules and adequate parametrization; they constitute the matter of
Sec. VII.

A. Processes of Drug Disposition

Bauer-Staeb and Niebes have measured the binding of polyphenols [ruto-side (I) and some of its O-β-hydroxyethyl derivatives] to human serum proteins [14]. Their results (Table 1) clearly indicate that the phenolic OH

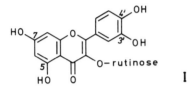

I

groups account for most of the binding, rather than the carbonyl groups and the several alcoholic OH groups (in the hydroxyethyl side chains and in the disaccharide). It is also apparent that a free catechol group affords the largest binding contribution, since the 4'-substitution decreases the binding by more than half.

The distribution of three aporphines into mouse brain has been studied by careful pharmacokinetic investigations [15]. The compounds are norapomorphine (the secondary amine), apomorphine (the N-methylated analog), and N-n-propylnorapomorphine; their concentration profiles in brain are shown in Fig. 1. The N-propyl and N-methyl derivatives appear to achieve immediate or very rapid (<5 min) brain/plasma equilibrium. Brain/plasma concentration ratios of 1/18.4 and 1/22.9, respectively, were achieved, whereas the highest observed brain contents (at 1 min) were 4.7% and 2.8%

TABLE 1
The binding of Polyphenols to Human Serum Proteins

Polyphenols	Degree of binding (% ± SD) at a drug concentration of 0.1 mg/ml
Rutoside (I)	70.9 ± 1.4
Mono-7-HR[a]	52.5 ± 2.7
Di-7,4'-HR	21.6 ± 2.7
Tri-7,3',4'-HR	11.6 ± 1.9
Tetra-5,7,3',4'-HR	5.4 ± 3.7

[a]HR = O-β-hydroxyethyl rutoside.
Source: From Ref. 14.

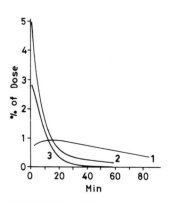

FIGURE 1   Time course in brain of norapomorphine (1), apomorphine (2), and N-n-propyl-apomorphine (3), following i.v. administration to mice. (From Ref. 15.)

of the dose, respectively. These results, although consistent with the higher lipophilicity of the N-propyl derivative, cannot be extrapolated in a straightforward manner to predict a decreased brain/plasma concentration ratio for the less lipophilic norapomorphine. Indeed, the latter drug showed a very slow distribution into brain, no brain/plasma equilibrium seemingly being reached. The resulting brain concentration profile (Fig. 1) thus cannot be compared with those of the two other compounds and suggests considerable differences (possibly of a qualitative nature) between the distribution of the secondary amine, on the one hand, and that of the tertiary amines, on the other. Such an example illustrates one of the great dangers encountered in studying structure-disposition relationships, namely, that of comparing results and data which are not comparable.

In another study, amphetamine (II) and its rigid analogs 2-aminoindan (III), 2-aminotetralin (IV), and 2-aminobenzocycloheptane (V) were determined following administration to rats [16] (Table 2). Pretreatment of animals with iprindole, an inhibitor of amphetamine aromatic hydroxylation, increases all half-lives two- to threefold (range, 3.3-3.9 hr). This finding indicates that all four drugs are metabolized by aromatic hydroxylation in the rat. The similarity of brain level profiles and distribution in various organs further suggests a comparable fate of the four compounds. In fact, the $t_{1/2}$ values are highly correlated ($r^2 = 0.988$) with the log P values (Table 2), which we have calculated according to Rekker [17]. The latter result means that the half-lives of the four amphetamines are accounted for almost exclusively by their hydrophobic properties. It would be tempting, therefore, to write down an equation correlating log P to $t_{1/2}$. However, because the correlation is based on only four observations and because the spread of $t_{1/2}$ values is very limited, such an equation has no extrapolative value and would fallaciously appear as sound. We conclude that the study

TABLE 2
Half-lives in Rat Brain of Amphetamine (II) and Some Rigid Analogs (III-V)

Structure	$t_{1/2}$ (hr)	log P [a]
II	1.4	1.99
III	1.7	1.63
IV	1.3	2.16
V	1.0	2.68

[a]Specifically, log P of the true octanol/water partition coefficient, calculated according to Rekker [17].
Source: From Ref. 16.

being discussed has allowed a qualitative understanding of the biological
and chemical factors governing the fate of amphetamine analogs in the rat.

B. Oxidative Pathways of Biotransformation

Reactions of oxidative dealkylation have been investigated using large series of substrates (ten or more); such studies can often be analyzed in terms of quantitative structure-metabolism relationships (to be discussed in Sec. VII).

A careful study of the rat liver microsomal N-demethylation of a series of aralkylamines as a function of pH has supplied a wealth of information on the kinetic aspects of this reaction [18]. The inhibitory effect of the proton on demethylation, expressed in terms of pK_i, were compared to pK_a values determined under conditions of identical temperature and ionic strength (Table 3). The pK_i and pK_a values of each compound would be identical if the reaction were to be described as a simple competition between proton and enzyme for the substrate (the un-ionized base). However, the pK_a and pK_i values differ, and the results were interpreted in terms of a model in which the rate of demethylation is dependent on two equilibria—the ionization of the base and its partition between the lipophilic microsomes

TABLE 3
Physical Properties and Microsomal N-Demethylation of Tertiary Aralkylamines

Aralkylamines	pK_a[a]	pK_i[b]	pK_a-pK_i	log P_{oct}[c]	log P_{hept}[a]
N-Dimethylbenzylamine	8.90	7.53	1.37	1.67	1.38
N-Dimethylphenylethylamine	9.17	7.65	1.52	2.20	1.39
N-Dimethylphenylpropylamine	9.43	7.43	2.04	2.73	1.84
N-Dimethylamphetamine	9.51	7.49	2.02	2.61	1.79
N-Dimethylphentermine	9.64	8.01	1.63	3.22	1.98

[a]As determined experimentally [18].
[b]Competitive inhibition by H^+ of the reaction of N-demethylation.
[c]Calculated according to Rekker [17].
Source: From Ref. 18.

and the aqueous incubation media. From such a model, the approximate Eq. (1) has been derived [18]:

$$pK_i = pK_a - \log P \tag{1}$$

Indeed, the experimental data agree reasonably well with this equation. In particular, the pK_a-pK_i differences are in most cases intermediate between the logarithms of the n-octanol/water and n-heptane/water partition coefficients.

Although the number of observations (i.e., the number of investigated compounds) is too small for a statistical evaluation of the data, this study has indicated in a qualitative but nevertheless conclusive manner that the two structural properties controlling the N-demethylation of the investigated compounds are their basicity and their ability to partition between aqueous media and microsomes.

The pathways of aromatic ring oxidation have similarly been investigated by using series of analogs as substrates. For example, the metabolism of 4,4'-dihalogenobiphenyls (VI) in the rabbit has led to the unambiguous characterization and quantification of three phenolic metabolites, namely, the 4-halogeno-3-hydroxy (VII), the 3-halogeno-4-hydroxy (VIII), and the 4-hydroxy (IX) derivatives [19]. The last two metabolites result from an NIH shift mechanism involving either retention (VIII) or loss (IX) of the halogen atom. Comparison of the fate of the three analogs (Table 4) shows that the NIH shift contribution decreases in the series of Cl-Br-I (50%-23%-0%). When the NIH shift takes place, it is accompanied by more loss than retention of the halogen atom; the relatively greater loss of chlorine as compared to bromine (3:1 versus 2:1) can hardly be considered significant.

In the complex field of N-oxide formation from tertiary amines, a semblance of order has emerged from a hypothesis formulated by Gorrod [20]. This author has divided nitrogen-containing moieties into three groups: groups I (basic amines, pK_a 8-11); group III (nonbasic nitrogen-containing groups); and the intermediate group II (weak bases, pK_a 1-7). A compilation of metabolic data led to the hypothesis that the group I amines are oxidized by flavin-cofactored monooxygenases, whereas group III compounds are oxidized by cytochrome-P-450-dependent systems. Compounds of group II appear as substrates for both enzyme systems, their relative contributions depending on a number of factors.

In this example, a global consideration of series of amines has allowed some insight into the nature of operating enzymes. Recent studies, however, have shown that basic tertiary amines are substrates for both classes of monooxygenases [e.g., 21], and this problem therefore calls for more investigations.

The oxidative dearylation of paraoxon analogs is a poorly understood reaction showing a very high and unusual substrate selectivity. In this case,

TABLE 4

Metabolism of 4,4'-Dihalogenobiphenyls (VI) in the Rabit

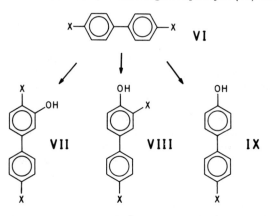

	Relative yield of urinary metabolites		
Substrate	VII	VIII	IX
X = Cl	4	1	3
X = Br	10	1	2
X = I	Sole metabolite	0	0

Source: From Ref. 19.

the substrate selectivity may well prove to be a major clue in assessing the mechanism of the reaction. The insecticide parathion (X) is oxidatively de-arylated by monooxygenases to yield as final products para-nitrophenol, diethylphosphoric acid, and diethylphosphorothioic acid (Scheme 1). The reaction is thought to be initiated by oxidative attack on the sulfur atom to yield a sulfine; the latter is readily hydrolyzed to liberate para-nitrophenol (for a review, see Ref. 22). The sulfine intermediate also yields the very toxic metabolite paraoxon (XI) via an oxathiaphosphirane intermediate.

Paraoxon is known to be degraded by nonoxidative dearylation cata-lyzed by A-esterases (route B in Scheme 1), resulting in the formation of diethylphosphoric acid and para-nitrophenol. On the other hand, paraoxon is not a substrate for the monooxygenase-catalyzed oxidative dearylation (route A in Scheme 1) which would result in a phosphorus derivative of un-known nature and para-nitrophenol. These facts have prompted Cammer

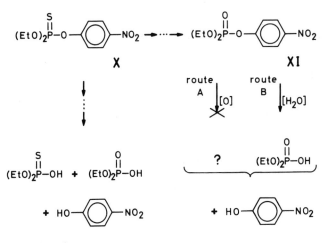

· SCHEME 1

and Hollingworth [23] to investigate the activity of paraoxon analogs as substrates for oxidative dearylation. The results (Table 5) show that several derivatives are good substrates for this reaction whereas others appear not to be substrates at all. Rationalizing these results in terms of structure-activity relationships reveals that with the exception of the 2-methoxyethyl derivative, all good substrates have at least one substituent possessing a three-atom chain, preferably a three-carbon chain. Failure to display this structural feature results in total or almost total lack of reactivity. Such a high substrate selectivity appears to be better explainable in terms of the mechanism of reaction rather than by enzyme affinity. Thus, turning our attention back to the mechanism of parathion (X) dearylation, a peroxide-type linkage analogous to the sulfine may be postulated for the oxidative intermediate of the paraoxon analogs. The question would then be: How does a three-atom chain facilitate the formation of a peroxide-type intermediate or divert its rearrangement toward hydrolytic cleavage of the ester bond? To answer this question, the authors of this study have proposed a rational mechanism, namely, oxidative $(\omega-1)$-attack at the β-carbon of derivatives XII to yield a hydroxylated derivative of structure XIII, followed by cyclization to a dioxaphospholane derivative (XIV) and expulsion of para-nitrophenol. The regioselectivity for the $(\omega-1)$ position (see Sec. IV) would explain the requirement for a three-carbon chain, whereas oxidative O-de-methylation of the 2-methoxyethyl substituent would yield an active 2-hydroxy-ethyl chain. Attempts to synthesize a dioxaphospholane derivative XIV have failed, thus precluding testing of the hypothesis. However, the failure to detect di-n-propyl phosphate and the known instability of phospholanes of structure XIV are compatible with the proposed mechanistic hypothesis [23].

TABLE 5

Oxidative Dearylation of Paraoxon Analogs by Mouse Liver Microsomes

$$\begin{array}{c} RO \\ \diagdown \\ O{=}P{-}O{-}(\text{p-nitrophenyl}) \\ \diagup \\ R'O \end{array}$$

Analog R = R'	V_{max} (nmol/mg/min)
Methyl	$--^a$
Ethyl	$--^b$
n-Propyl	30.0
Isopropyl	3.6
n-Butyl	$--^a$
s-Butyl	23.7
Isobutyl	35.6
n-Pentyl	$--^a$
Isopentyl	$--^a$
1-Ethylpropyl	21.9
2-Methylbutyl	17.8
2-Methoxyethyl	15.3
2-Chloroethyl	13.7
Allyl	21.7

Analog		V_{max} (nmol/mg/min)
R	R'	
Ethyl	n-Propyl	23.4
Ethyl	n-Butyl	$--^a$
n-Butyl	n-Propyl	15.5

[a] No production of para-nitrophenyl observed.
[b] Reaction rate: 1.0 nmol/mg/min, too low for the determination of V_{max}.
Source: From Ref. 23.

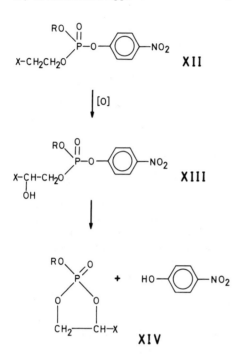

XII

XIII

XIV

C. Reductive and Hydrolytic Pathways

The recently reported liver microsomal nitroxide reduction catalyzed by cytochrome P-450 involves the transfer of one electron to the nitroxide to yield the corresponding hydroxylamino anion; it has been proposed that the ferrous form of the cytochrome donates the electron to the nitroxide and in turn is oxidized to the ferric state [24]. While 2,2,6,6-tetramethylpiperidinoxyl radical [(XV); TEMPO] is well reduced by liver microsomes, 2-ethyl-2,4,4-trimethyl-3-oxazolidinoxyl radical [(XVI); OXAN] is not. No

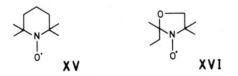

XV   **XVI**

electronic effect due to the ether oxygen is involved in this lack of reactivity since the two nitroxides possess the identical half-reduction potential of 300 mV, that is, below the reported reduction potential for cytochrome P-450 Fe^{2+} of 330 mV [25].

Microsomal preparations from 3-methylcholanthrene-induced rats again do not reduce OXAN. On the other hand, induction by phenobarbital results in an enzyme system very active toward both OXAN and TEMPO. Also of interest is the fact that in control rats OXAN is a competitive inhibitor of TEMPO bioreduction ($K_i = 7 \times 10^{-5}$ M). These findings indicate that OXAN binds to normal cytochrome P-450 at a site which does not allow electron transfer, but which prevents TEMPO binding. It would also appear that phenobarbital induces the synthesis of a new form of cytochrome P-450 whose active site topology must significantly differ from that of normal cytochrome since it allows a productive binding of OXAN [25]. The study being considered is therefore of considerable value in that it reveals a major difference between the active sites and the catalytic activities of two distinct cytochrome P-450's. Noteworthy is the fact that these conclusions were reached with the use of a very limited number of substrates.

Hydrolysis reactions are much studied in the development of prodrugs. An example is seen in the investigation of acyl-substituted mono- and diesters of terbutaline (XVII) with the goal of facilitating absorption from the gastrointestinal tract [26]. Human serum esterase (shown to be a single enzyme) catalyzes the hydrolysis of the investigated esters. The results reported in Table 6 show that the diesters hydrolyze to the monoesters at a slower rate than the rate at which the monoesters hydrolyze to terbutaline. This fact has been interpreted as indicating that the rate-limiting step in the reaction is not deacylation of the substrates, but rather acylation of the enzyme. Steric hindrance during the acylation reaction may be one of the reasons for the faster hydrolysis of the monoesters. From the values of V_{max} in Table 6 it is evident that increased branching and bulk of the acyl substituents decreases the rate of hydrolysis, whereas they do not seem to have any significant influence on the values of K_m. Such conclusions supply useful (even if not quantitative) information for the design of an optimal prodrug.

Fundamental mechanistic insight can be gained from quantum mechanical interpretation of metabolic results, as will be shown by a few examples in this chapter. An interesting case is provided by the NADPH-dependent dechlorination of chloroethane analogs by rat liver microsomes [27]; the metabolic results have prompted Loew and coworkers to calculate quantum mechanical parameters for the molecules being investigated [28]. Although the theoretical method used is cheap in terms of computer time and very daring in its approximations, usable indicative values are generally obtained. Bond strengths (C—Cl, C—C, C—H) and net atomic charges showed intermolecular variations which did not appear to be correlated with the observed extent of metabolic chlorination. On the other hand, a clear correlation was revealed with the degree of electron deficiency in the most electron-deficient carbon valence orbital (Table 7). Further, in every molecule this carbon orbital is involved exclusively in bonding to a chlorine atom [28]. These results indicate that the initial rate-determining step in the metabolic dechlorination is a nucleophilic attack on that carbon atom orbital. Such a mechanism is hydrolytic in nature, as opposed to known oxidative or reductive pathways of dehalogenation. The aforementioned

TABLE 6
Human Serum Esterase-Catalyzed Hydrolysis
of Mono- and Diesters of Terbutaline (XVII)

XVII

Terbutaline esters	$K_m{}^a$	$V_{max}{}^b$
Monoesters (R = H)		
R' = CH_3CO	4.9	98.6
R' = $(CH_3)_2CHCO$	2.3	89.2
Diesters[c]		
R = R' = CH_3CO	7.1	71.1
R = R' = CH_3CH_2CO	5.2	73.6
R = R' = $(CH_3)_2CHCO$	2.3	10.1
R = R' = $CH_3CH_2(CH_3)CHCO$	2.6	1.6
R = R' = $(CH_3)_3CCO$	4.8	0.17

[a] $M \times 10^5$
[b] $(mmol/sec) \times 10^5$
[c] The data refer to hydrolysis of diesters to monoesters.
Source: From Ref. 26.

results, however, would require confirmation by nonempirical (ab initio)
quantum mechanical methods before being accepted as genuinely reliable.

D. Reactions of Conjugation

As a general rule, conjugation reactions are genuine detoxification processes. This fact partly accounts for the great interest taken in these pathways and for the numerous studies devoted to them.
    One of the topics of current concern is the fate of metabolically pro-
duced epoxides, encompassing the factors that influence such parameters
as their stability, reactivity toward cellular components, detoxification or
toxification by epoxide hydrase, and detoxification by glutathione-S-epoxide
transferases. In this context, we now consider an important study in which
the reactivity of 45 epoxides (variously substituted oxiranes, XVIII-XXI,

TABLE 7
Dechlorination of Chloroethanes by Rat Liver Microsomes and Electron
Density in the Most Electron-Deficient Carbon Valence Orbital (f_+)

Molecule $C_\alpha - C_\beta$	Percentage of dechlorination	f_+ (carbon atom, valence atomic orbital)[a]
CH_3-CHCl_2	13.5	0.76 $(C_\beta, 2p_x)$
$CH_2Cl-CHCl_2$	9.8	0.77 $(C_\beta, 2p_y)$
$CHCl_2-CHCl_2$	6.0	0.78 $(2p_y)$
$CHCl_2-CCl_3$	1.7	0.79 $(C_\alpha, 2p_y)$
$CH_2Cl-CCl_3$	0.8	0.82 $(C_\beta, 2p_z)$
CH_3-CCl_3	<0.5	0.82 $(C_\beta, 2p_y, 2p_z)$
CH_3-CH_2Cl	<0.5	0.88 $(C_\beta, 2p_x)$
CH_2Cl-CH_2Cl	<0.5	0.89 $(2p_y)$
CCl_3-CCl_3	$(3.9)^b$	0.84 $(2p_x, 2p_y)$

[a] Calculated for the preferred conformation by the IEHT (iterative extended
Hückel theory) method.
[b] A dubious experimental result.
Source: Data from Refs. 27 and 28.

and arene oxides) toward sheep liver glutathione-S-epoxide transferase has
been investigated in an attempt to assess structural factors influencing this
reactivity [29,30]. The results for 19 selected oxiranes are compiled in
Table 8. Considering first the monosubstituted derivatives (Table 8, Part
A), the effect of lipophilicity is indicated by the lack of reactivity of the polar hydroxymethyl derivative as opposed to the relatively fast conjugation
of the more lipophilic chloromethyl derivatives. An opposite effect (de-
creasing reactivity with increasing lipophilicity) is however seen with styrene oxide and its halogenated derivatives (Table 8, Part A). This could
point to a parabolic relationship between reactivity and lipophilicity, if we
neglect electronic effects. The latter, however, must have an influence—
as indicated by the different behavior of para- and meta-substituted styrene
oxides, although the direction of this influence is unclear.

Steric effects are obvious when we consider the relative lack of reactivity of 1,1-disubstituted and 1,1,2-trisubstituted derivatives (Table 8,
Parts B and D, respectively). The 1,2-disubstituted derivatives (Table 8,
Part C), on the other hand, show good intrinsic reactivity, being strongly
influenced by stereochemical factors and by lipophilic properties. These
influences appear in the relative reactivity of the two trans- and

TABLE 8

Activity of a Purified Sheep Liver Glutathione-S-epoxide Transferase Toward Substituted Oxiranes

Oxiranes	Product formation relative to styrene oxide
(A) Monosubstituted oxiranes (XVIII)	
R = phenyl (styrene oxide)	100
R = para-nitrophenyl	60
R = meta-nitrophenyl	31
R = para-bromophenyl	55
R = meta-bromophenyl	41
R = meta-chlorophenyl	65
R = 4-biphenyl	6.7
R = CH_2OH	ND[a]
R = CH_2Cl	51
R = CCl_3	41
(B) 1,1-Disubstituted oxiranes (XIX)	
R = R' = phenyl	ND[a]
R = CH_3; R' = phenyl	4.4
(C) 1,2-Disubstituted oxiranes (XX)	
R = R' = phenyl (trans-configuration) (stilbene oxide)	5
R = CH_3; R' = phenyl (trans)	114
R = CH_3; R' = phenyl (cis)	22
R = CH_3; R' = $COOCH_2CH_3$ (trans)	59
(D) 1,1,2-Trisubstituted oxiranes (XXI)	
R = R" = CH_3; R' = phenyl (trans)	1.8
R = R" = CH_3; R' = phenyl (cis)	1.8
R = R' = CH_3; R" = phenyl	14

[a]Not detectable.
Source: From Ref. 29

cis-diastereoisomers, and in the moderate and high reactivity of stilbene oxide (more lipophilic) and ethyl butyrate-2,3-oxide (more hydrophilic), respectively.

Despite the considerable effort involved in the aforementioned study, the results have failed to give a clear insight into structure-reactivity relationships. However, far from being a failure, the absence of usable structural information reflects the complexity of the problem and calls for much additional work. It is an inviting challenge which no doubt will soon be met.

Jacobson compared the rates of acetylation of various aniline derivatives (XXII), using pigeon liver acetyl transferase [31], and demonstrated a more than 100-fold range of acetylation rates (Table 9). As a general trend, the rate was found to decrease with increasing electronegativity of the substituent, but such an interpretation ignores the high reactivity of the halogenated derivatives. If one looks at solubility factors, however, another trend appears. Indeed, all derivatives which are more readily acetylated than aniline bear substituents that increase their lipophilicity as compared to the latter. On the other hand, all hydrophilic substituents (including the slightly hydrophilic nitro group; see Ref. 17) markedly decrease the reactivity of the substrate. Such a study therefore leads to the qualitative conclusion that hydrophilic—and perhaps also electronegative—substituents decrease the rate of acetylation of aniline derivatives by the test enzyme system. Only dubious extrapolations can be made as to the reactivity of other derivatives. The study is nevertheless of interest because it shows that the reactivity of various substrates may differ considerably, and because several of the investigated compounds pertain to medicinal chemistry (i.e., para-aminohippuric acid, sulfanilamide, para-aminosalicylic acid, para-aminobenzoic acid).

E. Induction of Drug-Metabolizing Enzymes

The qualitative structural approach discussed in Sec. II has further proved its value in studies of enzyme induction and inhibition. Examples considering induction by biphenyl derivatives will illustrate this point.

Using chick embryos, the efficacy of halogenated biphenyls (XXIII) in inducing hepatic aryl hydroxylase activity (a cytochrome-P-448-mediated activity) has been investigated [32]. The results (Table 10, Part A) reveal two structural requirements for activity, namely, the presence of at least two adjacent halogen atoms in the lateral positions of each benzene ring (positions 3,4,3',4' or 3,4,5,3',4',5') and the absence of halogen atoms adjacent to the biphenyl bridge. The first requirement is presumably related to adequate lipophilicity and molecular area. The second requirement was taken to

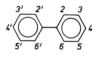

XXIII

TABLE 9
Relative Rates of Acetylation of Aniline Derivatives
by Pigeon Liver Acetyl Transferase

H_2N—⟨benzene ring⟩—R   **XXII**
                        R'

Substrate (XXII)	Relative rate
R = R' = H	70
R = CH_3; R' = H	100
R = Cl; R' = H	109
R = Br; R' = H	112
R = NO_2; R' = H	34
R = $CONHCH_2COOH$; R' = H	25
R = SO_2NH_2; R' = H	18
R = COOH; R' = OH	15
R = COOH; R' = H	3
R = SO_2OH; R' = H	1

Source: From Ref. 31.

indicate that coplanarity or near-coplanarity of the two rings is a prerequisite for activity, since substituents at the ortho positions lead to marked
nonplanarity of the molecule.

The hypothesis of a planarity factor has been verified using biphenylene
derivatives (XXIV). In this limited series the substitution-activity pattern
(Table 10, Part B) follows that of the biphenyl derivatives. On the other
hand, the full planarity of the biphenylenes renders them over 100 times
more potent than the somewhat flexible and not fully planar biphenyls. It is
interesting to note that the two active halogenated biphenylenes are roughly
equipotent with the well-known inducer 2,3,7,8-Tetra-chlorodibenzo-para-
dioxin (TCDD) [(XXV); Table 10, Part C]. The latter, rather than being fully planar, resembles a butterfly whose wings are not in the same plane.
However, this deviation from planarity is small (ca. 40°) and occurs along
the secondary molecular axis rather than along the principal axis in contrast
to the biphenyls.

The results of the foregoing study are complementary to the data produced in an examination [33] of a number of chlorinated biphenyls as inducers

TABLE 10

Potency of Biphenyls and Structural Analogs in Inducing Hepatic Aryl Hydrocarbon Hydroxylase Activity in Chick Embryos

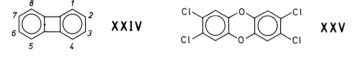

Biphenyls and analogs	ED_{50} (nmol/kg)
(A) Halogenated biphenyls (XXIII)	
Biphenyl	ND^a
4-Cl	ND
3,4-Cl$_2$	ND
4,4'-Cl$_2$	ND
2,6,2',6'-Cl$_4$	ND
2,4,3',4'-Cl$_4$	ND
2,3,2',3'-Cl$_4$	ND
3,5,3',5'-Cl$_4$	ND
3,5,3',5'-Br$_4$	ND
3,4,3',4'-Cl$_4$	88
3,4,5,3',4',5'-Cl$_6$	94
3,4,5,3',4',5'-Br$_6$	68
2,3,4,2',3',4'-Cl$_6$	ND
2,4,5,2',4',5'-Cl$_6$	ND
2,4,6,2',4',6'-Cl$_6$	ND
Cl$_{10}$	ND
(B) Biphenylene derivatives (XXIV)	
2,3,6,7-Cl$_4$	0.28
2,3,6,7-Br$_4$	0.44
Cl$_8$	ND
2,7-(NO$_2$)$_2$	ND
2,3,6,7-(OCH$_3$)$_4$	ND
(C) Dibenzo-para-dioxin derivative	
TCDD (XXV)	0.2

[a]Not detectable.

Source: From Ref. 32.

of various hepatic enzyme systems, for example, aryl hydrocarbon hydroxylase (AHH; cytochrome P-448-mediated; 3-methylcholanthrene inducible); aminopyrine N-demethylase (APND; cytochrome P-450 mediated; phenobarbital inducible), glycyronyltransferase, and the terminal oxidase cytochrome P-450. From the results (Table 11) it can be seen that only two derivatives are extremely potent AHH inducers, namely, 3,4,3',4'-tetrachloro- and 3,4,5,3',4',5'-hexachlorobiphenyl (as also seen in Table 10). However, these two derivatives differentially alter APND, since the former is without effect and the latter is a potent inhibitor; they also differ in their effects on glucuronyltransferase. On the other hand, this work shows that some weak-to-moderate inducers of AHH are relatively good inducers of APND and cytochrome P-450. These biphenyls are characterized by being chlorinated in the 2,4,2',4'-positions, regardless of the chlorination of the meta positions. This structural requirement contrasts with the prerequisite for strong AHH induction, namely, no 2-substituent, suggesting topological differences in the "receptor" sites. In particular, it would appear that planarity is not a structural requirement for a molecule to act as a cytochrome P-450 inducer (phenobarbital is not a planar molecule). Indeed, it may even be assumed that planarity is incompatible with cytochrome P-450 induction.

Summarizing the structure-activity relationships for induction by halogenated biphenyls, it appears as a first approximation that occupation of the two para positions is important for activity. Substitution at both meta and para positions induces cytochrome P-448. Further substitution at ortho positions decreases or abolishes this activity but results in cytochrome P-450 induction

F. Overview

In this section we have discussed a number of examples showing how broadly understood factors can influence substrate selectivity in drug metabolism. The examples are pertinent to various aspects of drug disposition and to various metabolic routes. Several aspects of structure-metabolism relationships have been illustrated by the selected examples:

Influence of functional groups on protein binding (Table 1)
Influence of homology and lipophilicity on disposition (Fig. 1; Table 2)
Influence of ionization and lipophilicity on microsomal uptake and
    metabolism (Table 3)
Influence of substituents on mechanisms of biotransformation (Tables
    4 and 5)
Influence of substituents on reaction rates (Tables 5, 6, 7, 8, and 9)
The role of substituents in helping to assess reaction mechanisms
    (Tables 5 and 7)
The role of analogous substrates as a tool in investigation of enzymic
    properties (Tables 6, 10, and 11)

TABLE 11
Relative Activity of Chlorinated Biphenyls (XXIII) as Inducers
of Drug-Metabolizing Enzymes in Female Weaning Rats[a]

Inducer	AHH[b]	APND[c]	Glucuronyl-transferase
Control (corn oil)	100	100	100
Biphenyl	80^d	90^d	110^d
$2,2'\text{-Cl}_2$	100^d	120^d	120^d
$3,3'\text{-Cl}_2$	110^d	110^d	120^d
$4,4'\text{-Cl}_2$	150^d	140^d	100^d
$2,4\text{-Cl}_2$	120^d	110^d	120^d
$2,3,2',3'\text{-Cl}_4$	190	130^d	100^d
$2,4,2',4'\text{-Cl}_4$	200	170	100^d
$3,4,3',4'\text{-Cl}_4$	3500	90^d	300
$3,5,3',5'\text{-Cl}_4$	230	120^d	100^d
$2,6,2',6'\text{-Cl}_4$	140^d	120^d	110^d
$2,5,2',5'\text{-Cl}_4$	140^d	120^d	100^d
$2,3,4,5\text{-Cl}_4$	210	100^d	90^d
$2,3,5,6\text{-Cl}_4$	160	110^d	90^d
$2,5,3',4'\text{-Cl}_4$	130^d	100^d	120^d
$2,3,6,2',3',6'\text{-Cl}_6$	110^d $(60^{d,e})$	90^d $(90^{d,e})$	100^d $(100^{d,e})$
$2,3,4,2',3',4'\text{-Cl}_6$	580	200	200
$2,4,5,2',4',5'\text{-Cl}_6$	330 $(140^{d,e})$	250 (190^e)	120^d $(110^{d,e})$
$2,4,6,2',4',6'\text{-Cl}_6$	190 $(100^{d,e})$	150^d (130^e)	110^d $(110^{d,e})$
$3,4,5,3',4',5'\text{-Cl}_6$	900 (2100^e)	30 (60^e)	20 (200^e)

[a] All reported results were obtained at a 140 nmol/kg dosage level unless
otherwise indicated.
[b] Aryl hydrocarbon hydroxylase, a cytochrome-P-448-mediated activity.
[c] Aminopyrine N-demethylase, a cytochrome-P-450-mediated activity.
[d] Value not statistically different ($P > 0.05$) from control.
[e] Result obtained at a 30 nmol/kg dosage level.
Source: From Ref. 33.

Some of the examples lead to interesting conclusions; others seemingly do not. In all cases, however, nothing more than qualitative interpretations are possible. This situation will also prevail in the following sections, in which structural factors pertaining to constitutional isomerism and stereoisomerism will be considered. Only in Sec. VII will the concepts of parametrization and quantitative structure-activity relationships be applied to drug disposition in order to demonstrate that a jump from qualitative to quantitative conclusions may be achieved under favorable conditions.

III. SUBSTRATE REGIO- AND STEREOSELECTIVITY

The conventional classification of structural isomers (chemical species having the same molecular formula) is based upon bonding connectivity, i.e., the pattern of bonding connection of atoms in a molecule. As a result, a discrimination is made between isomers which are identically connected (stereoisomers) and those which are not (constitutional isomers). Classification according to symmetry then divides stereoisomers into enantiomers and diastereoisomers [34].

This categorization, although unambiguous and widely accepted, is not fully satisfactory, as demonstrated by Mislow [35]. Indeed, enantiomers have identical physical and chemical properties, whereas diastereoisomers differ in every chemical and physical property, however small the difference. As such, diastereoisomers resemble constitutional isomers more than enantiomers. Instead of considering the sole bonding connectivity of atoms in a molecule, Mislow takes into account pairwise interrelationships between all atoms, connected or nonconnected. Suitable pairwise interrelationships are, for example, interatomic distances. Structural isomers having identical sets of pairwise interrelationships are said to be isometric; otherwise, they are anisometric. Isometric molecules are homomeric (identical) or enantiomeric, depending on whether they are superimposable or not. Anisometric molecules are diastereoisomeric or constitutionally isomeric, depending on whether their atoms are identically connected or not. Such a classification has the merit of placing in one category (that of the isometric molecules) isomers which have identical chemical and physical properties (in our context enantiomers) and in a distinct category (that of anisometric molecules) isomers having different properties (diastereoisomers and constitutional isomers) [34].

The foregoing classification has been discussed at some length since it provides a useful approach to substrate selectivity, which implies that one isomeric form is preferentially removed as compared to the other(s)[*].

---

[*]But without the introduction of additional elements of isomerism (e.g., creation of a center of chirality), in which case we would have a situation of substrate-product regio- or stereoselectivity. In the case of substrate selectivity, the biotransformation can occur either with retention or with loss of the element(s) of isomerism.

In the case of anisometric isomers, differential disposition or biotransformation may or may not be of enzymic origin since differences in physical properties may account for the selectivity. For example, variations in the concentration of substrates entering the enzymic phase may be due to differences in lipophilicity. On the other hand, the discrimination between enantiomers in terms of substrate stereoselectivity necessitates a chiral handle (an enzyme, or even a chiral constituent of the chiral biological environment). Thus, when two enantiomers bind to an enzyme, two diastereoisomeric complexes are formed which differ in such properties as stability and transition state energy. From this discussion it is clear that a marked conceptual difference exists in the substrate selectivities of isometric and anisometric molecules. This conceptual difference is of great practical significance in drug disposition (absorption, distribution, excretion) where interactions with enzymes or other chiral biomolecules are not necessarily involved. If such interactions do not take place, anisometric substrates may behave differently whereas enantiomers will not; if they do occur, substrate selectivity exists but may escape detection.

In drug binding and biotransformation, chiral macromolecules or enzymes are necessarily involved and substrate selectivity (observable or not) is the rule for all structural isomers.

A schematic summary of the preceding discussion is given in Table 12. Several conceivable situations are presented, some of which will be encountered in the various examples to be discussed in this section.

A. Drug Disposition and Binding of Enantiomers

Not infrequently, profiles of plasma drug concentration versus time are published that show differences in the behavior of enantiomers. For example, the plasma half-lives of the amphetamine (L) enantiomers show considerable differences under various experimental conditions (Table 13), the (R)-(-)-isomer always disappearing at a slower rate [36]. Such results when considered alone are not very informative since they allow no conclusion as to the origin of the observed elimination selectivity. Only in the general context of our knowledge does it become clear that selective biotransformation often accounts for the differences in half-lives [5], as will be discussed later.

Detailed pharmacokinetic investigations may be more informative than simple half-life determinations, but the number and complexity of intermingling basic processes tend to blur the interpretation of individual phenomena. This is illustrated by the fate of the anticoagulant drugs phenprocoumon (XXVI) and warfarin (XXVII) in rats and humans. From a compilation of some pharmacokinetic parameters (Table 14), it is readily apparent that the differences between the (R)- and (S)-enantiomers are either nonexistent, dubious, or not considerable when at all statistically significant. The mean values for both isomers often display a large standard deviation

TABLE 12
Phenomena Underlying Substrate Selectivity of Structural Isomers in Drug Metabolism and Disposition

	Drug disposition (absorption, distribution, excretion)		Drug binding		Biotransformation	
	ANISO[a]	ISO[b]	ANISO[a]	ISO[b]	ANISO[a]	ISO[b]
Differences in physico-chemical properties	yes	no	yes	no	yes	no
Interaction with chiral biomolecules	yes or no	yes or no	yes	yes	yes or no	yes or no
Enzymic reactions	yes or no	yes or no	no	no	yes	yes
Overall substrate selectivity[c]	yes	yes or no	yes	yes	yes	yes

[a]ANISO: anisometric substrates (diastereoisomers and constitutional isomers).
[b]ISO: isometric substrates (enantiomers).
[c]Substrate selectivity may escape experimental detection by being too small or obscured by other phenomena.

TABLE 13
Plasma Half-Lives of Amphetamine (A) Enantiomers Measured
in a Single Human Volunteer under Various Conditions

	$t_{1/2}$ (hr)		
Conditions	(S)-(+)	(R)-(-)	R/S ratio
Acidic urine (pH 5.05-7.53) 10 mg (±)-A	5.9	6.8	1.15
Alkaline urine (pH 6.71-8.03) 10 mg (±)-A	15.2	23.6	1.55
Alkaline urine (pH 6.70-8.14) 10 mg (+)-A or (-)-A on separate occasions	13.1	30.1	2.3

Source: From Ref. 36.

owing to interindividual variations which obscure assessment of differences.
This difficulty is partly overcome by considering the R/S ratio for each subject and calculating mean values. Values obtained for the racemates lie between those of the enantiomers when the latter show some differences.

The two main factors influencing the plasma half-lives of phenprocoumon and warfarin enantiomers are their binding to serum proteins and biotransformation. Only the first factor, protein binding, is taken into account
in the pharmacokinetic studies reported in Table 14. Extensive pharmacokinetic modeling would be required to approach a quantitative assessment of
metabolic disposition. On the other hand, the data in Table 14 indicate that
the enantioselective pharmacological activity of the two drugs is only mar-
ginally dependent upon pharmacokinetic differences. Indeed, the two (S)-
isomers are four to six times more potent than their (R)-enantiomers in the
rat, and two to three times more potent in human subjects.

Stereoselective binding to serum proteins as exemplified in Table 14
is a classical and well-documented phenomenon which will not be considered
further here. Of more recent interest is the growing awareness that uptake
of drugs by various organs may be enantioselective and thus differences in
uptake may not simply parallel differences in plasma concentrations. For
example, the liver/plasma concentration ratios of (S)-(-)- and (R)-(+)-phen-
procoumon in the rat were found to be statistically different, the values being 6.9 ± 0.5 and 5.2 ± 0.2, respectively [38], indicating a preferred uptake
of the more potent enantiomer.

TABLE 14

Pharmacokinetic Parameters of the (R)-(+)- and (S)-(-)-Enantiomers of Phenprocoumon (XXVI) and Warfarin (XXVII) in Rats and Humans

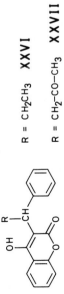

$R = CH_2CH_3$ **XXVI**

$R = CH_2{-}CO{-}CH_3$ **XXVII**

	Phenprocoumon				Warfarin			
	(RS)	(R)	(S)	R/S[a]	(RS)	(R)	(S)	R/S[a]
Plasma half-lives (hr ± SD)								
Rat	15.0 ± 1.7	17.8 ± 1.8	12.5 ± 1.2[b]	--	--	8.6 ± 1.6	15.4 ± 2.8[b]	--
Human	132 ± 9	120 ± 5	122 ± 7	0.99 ± 0.03	42 ± 2	58 ± 5	33 ± 4[b]	--
Human	--	111 ± 27	144 ± 56	0.83 ± 0.29	--	45 ± 13	32 ± 13	1.45 ± 0.26
Distribution volumes (ml/kg)								
Rat	411 ± 27	406 ± 20	403 ± 24	--	--	not different		--
Human	131 ± 12	141 ± 5	114 ± 5	1.23 ± 0.14	113 ± 6			
Human	--	98 ± 20	88 ± 15	1.14 ± 0.27	--	104 ± 17	109 ± 13	0.96 ± 0.12
Protein binding (free concentration in serum as percentage of total concentration)								
Rat	0.97 ± 0.05	1.13 ± 0.06	0.76 ± 0.07[b]	--	1.07 ± 0.65	1.31 ± 0.84	0.84 ± 0.49	1.56 ± 0.35
Human	0.39 ± 0.03	0.56 ± 0.03	0.29 ± 0.09[b]	--	1.04 ± 0.35	1.18 ± 0.40	0.90 ± 0.32	1.32 ± 0.26

[a] Mean ± SD of R/S ratios for each subject.

[b] Statistically significant difference between (R)- and (S)-enantiomers.

Source: Compiled from Refs. 37–43.

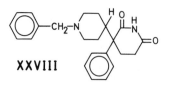

XXVIII

Another illustration of selective uptake is seen with the antimuscarinic drug benzetimide (XXVIII), whose pharmacologically potent (S)-(+)-enantiomer is selectively taken up into guinea pig cardiac tissues. The cardiac accumulation was found to be almost entirely due to nonspecific binding. The nonspecific binding sites therefore display a certain stereoselectivity—but to a much smaller extent than the pharmacological receptor binding sites [44].

The foregoing example illustrates the relevance of selective tissue binding, particularly when that tissue contains the receptor phase. Another example is provided by the β-adrenergic blocking agent propranolol (XXIX).

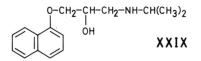

XXIX

Following intravenous administration of the racemate to rats, the serum and heart concentrations of the individual enantiomers were monitored. After 5 min, the serum levels of the pharmacologically active (S)-(-)-form were three times lower than those of its enantiomer. During the following 4 hr however, the (+)-form disappeared much faster from the serum (half-life 23.8 min) than the (-)-form (52.0 min). The initially lower levels of the (-)-form are explained by a highly selective cardiac uptake: most of the propranolol found in the heart was the (-)-isomer (82 ± 3% up to 90 min; ca. 100% after 2 hr). It thus appears that the active enantiomer is selectively accumulated in its organ of action, whereas the (R)-(+)-isomer remains in the blood and is stereoselectively and rapidly metabolized [45].

Stereoselective uptake of (-)-propranolol has also been found in the heart and brain of mice [46]. Furthermore, the statistically different plasma half-lives of (-)- and (+)-propranolol in man (3.20 ± 0.42 and 2.02 ± 0.53 hr) [47] closely parallel the rat values, suggesting a comparable selective cardiac uptake.

An interesting case of stereoselective liver uptake and enantiomeric interaction has been documented for propoxyphene (XXX). Only the

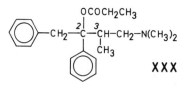

XXX

(2S;3R)-(+)-isomer shows analgesic activity in the rat. Strangely enough, a 20 mg/kg dose of this isomer in the rat is equiactive with a combination of the two enantiomers (2S;3R)-(+) and (2R;3S)-(-) (also designated dextro- and levo-propoxyphene, respectively) at a dose of 10 mg/kg each. The explanation for this synergistic effect was found in the disposition of the two enantiomers. When dextro-propoxyphene was infused in the isolated perfused rat liver, over 98% of the drug was extracted in a single pass; when levo-propoxyphene was added to the perfusate at the same concentration, the extraction of the dextro-isomer was decreased to less than 90%. A similar situation prevails in vivo, where the plasma levels of dextro-propoxyphene increased severalfold upon simultaneous dosing of its enantiomer. It therefore appears that levo-propoxyphene must be preferentially bound to uptake and/or metabolic sites within the liver, resulting in the release of dextro-propoxyphene into the systemic circulation and hence its increased systemic availability [48].

B. Regio- and Stereoselectivity in Overall Metabolism

Until now, substrate regioselectivity, that is, the comparative metabolism of separate regioisomers, has been paid only limited attention and treated in an empirical manner [11]. However, the examples available can often yield a wealth of mechanistic and enzymic information if thoroughly interpreted.

For instance, toluene-4-sulfonamide (XXXI) undergoes oxidation to 4-sulfamoylbenzoic acid (XXXII) in several species, as is usual in the metabolism of methylbenzenes. On the other hand, the metabolic fate of its

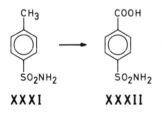

XXXI   **XXXII**

regioisomer toluene-2-sulfonamide (XXXIII), an impurity of commercial saccharin, has remained unknown. Recently, a study of the metabolism of the two isomers in the rat showed that, while XXXI was recovered mainly as XXXII, toluene-2-sulfonamide was metabolized predominantly by aromatic ring hydroxylation, the main metabolite (about two-thirds of the dose) being a phenol (XXXIV) excreted both free and as the glucuronide; less than 3% was oxidized to 2-sulfamoylbenzoic acid [49].

The two regioisomers are thus substrates for two distinct metabolic routes with a high degree of selectivity. The limited methyl oxidation of XXXIII can be postulated as being partly due to a steric hindrance effect of

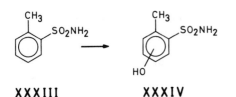

XXXIII   **XXXIV**

the sulfonamide moiety. On the other hand, the considerable ring oxidation of XXXIII is rather unexpected considering the known deactivating effect of the electron-withdrawing sulfonamide substituent (see Ref. 10). Predictably, the 4-position should be the least deactivated. However, unknown factors appear to be operative since a seemingly unfavorable reaction competes with an efficient metabolic route. New discoveries are needed in order to understand the factors accounting for this situation.

The in vivo metabolism of the three isomeric formylbenzoic acids [(XXXV), R = COOH] and of the three isomeric formylphenoxyacetic acids [(XXXV), R = OCH$_2$COOH] in several species is highly structure dependent [50]. It is indeed apparent from Table 15 that derivatives having a carboxylic group in the ortho position (phthalaldehydic acid and ortho-formylphenoxyacetic acid) are essentially reduced to the corresponding benzyl alcohol derivatives (XXXVI). The only real exception to this rule is the apparently predominant oxidation of ortho-formyl phenoxyacetic acid in the mouse; this may not be significant, however, since the reduced metabolite is further metabolized by alternate routes.

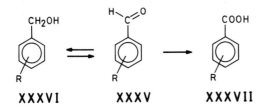

XXXVI   **XXXV**   **XXXVII**

On the other hand, the meta- and para-substituted aldehydes are essentially oxidized to diacids (XXXVII) with little or no competitive reduction. This can be simply expressed by saying that a qualitative difference exists in the metabolism of the ortho-isomers, on the one hand, and of the meta- and para-isomers, on the other. Such a difference is intriguing and calls for a tentative explanation. By the use of molecular models, it can be seen that an intramolecular hydrogen bond exists in the ortho derivative, phthalaldehydic acid (XXXVIII). Such an H-bond will influence the electron distribution within the carbonyl group by somewhat stabilizing a zwitterionic form (XXXVIII). As a result, the reactivity of the formyl group is modified in two ways: (1) the aldehyde reductase-catalyzed transfer of a hydride anion from NAD(P)H to the carbonyl carbon is facilitated by the increased electrophilic

TABLE 15
Effect of a Carbonyl Substituent on the Metabolism of Aromatic Aldehydes (XXXV) After Oral Administration

| | Aldehyde group metabolized to (percentage of dose): | | | | | | | |
| | Rat | | Mouse | | Rabbit | | Dog | |
Substrate	CH_2OH	COOH	CH_2OH	COOH	CH_2OH	COOH	CH_2OH	COOH
Formylbenzoic acids								
R = ortho-COOH	86	ND[a]	69	ND	69	ND	75	ND
meta-COOH	ND	97	--	--	--	--	ND	88
para-COOH	ND	87	--	--	--	--	ND	75
Formylphenoxyacetic acids								
R = ortho-OCH_2COOH	88	<2	15	35	57	<5	52	<2
meta-OCH_2COOH	24	79	--	--	--	--	--	--
para-OCH_2COOH	8	85	--	--	--	--	--	--

[a] ND: not detected.
Source: From Ref. 50.

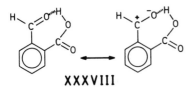

XXXVIII

character of that carbon; (2) the aldehyde dehydrogenase-catalyzed removal of the formyl hydrogen atom as a hydride anion is rendered more difficult by the increased partial positive charge on the carbonyl carbon. These two effects are expected to act synergistically in favoring bioreduction of the ortho derivatives.

It can be noted that the formation of an intramolecular H-bond is also feasible in ortho-formylphenoxyacetic acid (XXXIX). Such an H-bond, how-ever, is expected to be somewhat less strong than in XXXVIII due to the conformational freedom of the chain, and as a result the substrate regio-selectivity is not as high as with phthalaldehydic acid.

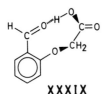

XXXIX

The two preceding examples have been selected because they illustrate how the study of regioisomeric substrates may give some insight into mech-anisms of enzymic reaction at the molecular level. Several other examples are known (e.g., the contrasted metabolism of L-3-O-methyldopa and L-4-O-methyldopa [51]) which can yield similar information on the nature and properties of the enzymes involved.

Substrate stereoselectivity is well documented [5, 52]; the selected studies discussed next will illustrate some uses and limits of investigation in studying stereoisomeric substrates.

Etomidate (XL) is an hypnotic agent whose activity resides in the (R)-(+)-enantiomer. The metabolism of both enantiomers has been investi-gated in vitro [53] and in vivo [54]. From these studies a tentative metabolic scheme can be drawn (Scheme 2) from which it appears that etomidate is metabolized by two competitive routes. Route A is initiated by ester hydroly-sis, whereas route B starts from N-dealkylation (postulated here to result from C_α-hydroxylation).

Urinary metabolite data (Table 16) show that (R)-(+)-etomidate is a better substrate for hydrolysis than is its enantiomer. On the other hand, more route B metabolites are generated from (S)-(-)- than from (R)-(+)-etomidate; this result is confirmed by the in vitro experiments—two of the

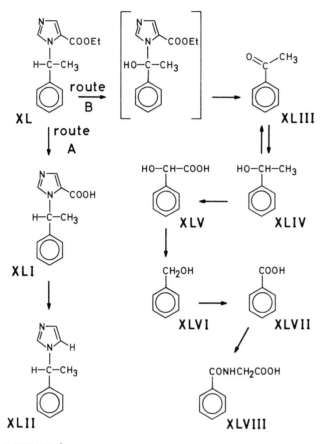

SCHEME 2

metabolites drawn in Scheme 2 [acetophenone (XLIII) and benzoic acid (XLVII)] being detected after incubations of (S)-etomidate only. An initial conclusion from this study would be that two competitive metabolic routes show opposed substrate stereoselectivity. However, another possible but unproven interpretation would be that route B is selective for (S)-etomidate simply because more (S)- than (R)-etomidate is available for N-dealkylation owing to the preferred hydrolytic removal of the latter enantiomer.

A comparable situation involving two competitive routes is encountered in the metabolism of 5-ethyl-3-methyl-5-phenylhydantoin (mephenytoin; XLIX) [55]. In the dog, the plasma levels of (-)-mephenytoin are higher than those of (+)-mephenytoin following separate administration of enantiomers. Similarly, more of the N-demethylated metabolite (ethotoin) is found in plasma and urine after administration of (-)- than (+)-mephenytoin.

TABLE 16
Excretion (over 24 hr) of Etomidate Metabolites in the Rat

	Percentage of administered dose	
	(R)-(+)-Etomidate	(S)-(-)-Etomidate
Total excretion in urine	76.7	75.8
Total excretion in the feces	10.5	8.9
Urinary metabolites:		
Etomidate acid (XLI)		
free	71.3	47.7
conjugated	3.0	4.4
Total route A	74.3	52.1
Mandelic acid (XLV)	2.4	6.3
Benzoic acid (XLVII)	1.6	2.8
Hippuric acid (XLVIII)	0.0	0.2
Total route B	4.0	9.3

Source: From Ref. 54.

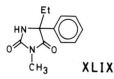

XLIX

The reverse holds for aryl-oxidized metabolites of unknown structure detected in urine. The reaction of aromatic oxidation of mephenytoin is characterized by a low apparent K_m value (high affinity of the substrate for the
substrate-enzyme complex), whereas the reaction of N-demethylation ex-
hibits a high K_m (low affinity of the substrate for the substrate-enzyme
complex). On the other hand, all results were found to be consistent with
a high and a low stereoselectivity for the reactions of aromatic oxidation
and N-demethylation, respectively. The correlation between enzyme affinity and degree of stereoselectivity is of great interest since it is consistent with Pfeiffer's rule [56], which states that high and low stereoselectivity

for drug-receptor interactions are the corrollaries of high and low affinities, respectively [55].

One of the most studied drugs with regards to its metabolism is amphetamine (L). The overall stereoselectivity of its metabolism in various species (Table 17) shows marked variation without apparent explanation. Indeed, the major metabolic route(s) in each species, when known, do not explain the observed variations in stereoselectivity. This would suggest as a first approximation that the same metabolic route can show different stereoselectivities (or no stereoselectivity) depending on the species [5].

The results of a classical study describing the metabolism of amphetamine enantiomers in the rat (Table 18) show that ring oxidation is the major route of amphetamine metabolism in this species [57]. The results also suggest (R)-(-)-amphetamine to be a better substrate than its enantiomer; alternatively, (+)-para-hydroxyamphetamine may be metabolized more readily than the (-)-isomer. Such a study therefore is of value in that it unravels useful information, but questions are left unanswered. Some of the answers may be obtained from the investigation of individual metabolic routes, as outlined in Sec. III.C.

By monitoring several major metabolites, in vitro studies in the rabbit have allowed a coherent and ample view of amphetamine metabolism in this species. Separate incubation of (R)-(-)- and (S)-(+)-amphetamine showed the former isomer to be a better substrate than its enantiomer for the two

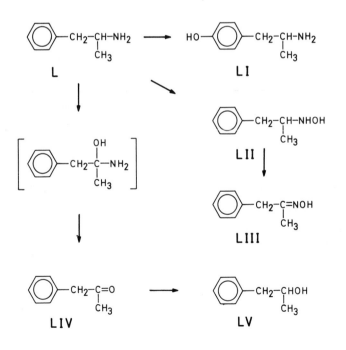

TABLE 17
Species Variation in the Stereoselectivity
of Overall Amphetamine Metabolism

Species	Stereoselectivity
Guinea pig	$S > R$
Rabbit	$S < R$
Sheep	$S > R$
Cattle	$S \equiv R$
Horse	$S > R$
Mouse	$S \equiv R$
Rat	$S \equiv R$
Swine	$S \equiv R$
Rhesus monkey	$S \equiv R$
Human	$S > R$

Source: Compilation from Ref. 5.

TABLE 18
Urinary Excretion of Amphetamine Metabolites in the Rat

| Metabolite | Percentage of dose | | |
	($\pm$)	(S)-(+)	(R)-(-)
Amphetamine (L)	13	12	17
para-Hydroxyamphetamine (LI)	60	48	63
Benzyl methyl ketone (LIV)	0	0	0
1-Phenyl-2-propanol (LV)	0	0	0
Benzoic acid	3	2	2
Total	76	62	82
^{14}C in urine	84	85	80

Source: From Ref. 57.

major pathways of deamination and N-oxidation [as assessed respectively by the formation of two major metabolites, 1-phenyl-2-propanol (LV) and N-hydroxyamphetamine (LII)]; see Table 19 [58]. Table 19 also shows that the concentration of (R)-N-hydroxyamphetamine produced from (R)-amphetamine decreased from the first to the third hour. The origin of this decrease was uncovered by incubations of the enantiomers of N-hydroxyamphetamine (LII) showing this metabolite to be metabolized to phenylacetone oxime (LIII) with a clear substrate stereoselectivity for the (R)-enantiomer (Table 19).

On the other hand, the results obtained with racemic amphetamine (Table 19) do not appear to agree with the findings for the individual enantiomers. As a first approximation it could be said that racemic amphetamine is metabolized as if the (R)-enantiomer were absent from the mixture, that is, as if the metabolism of this enantiomer were drastically inhibited [58]. This hypothesis has been verified by measuring the R/S ratios of metabolites formed after incubation of the separate enantiomers of amphetamine or the racemic modification (Table 20). The inhibition of the two pathways of (R)-amphetamine metabolism by its enantiomer (or one of its metabolites) is particularly striking; these results demonstrate that (S)-(+)-amphetamine, although less rapidly C_α- and N-hydroxylated than its enantiomer, has a greater affinity for the enzyme systems involved [59].

C. Regio- and Stereoselectivity in Individual
    Functionalization Reactions

Several interesting examples are known where regioisomeric compounds show substrate selectivity toward a particular drug-metabolizing enzyme system. Thus, fomocain (LVI, para-isomer) and its ortho-isomer undergo monooxygenase-mediated O-dealkylation resulting in the liberation of phenol. The reaction has been studied using rabbit liver preparations and shown to be markedly structure dependent [60]. Indeed, the K_m values for the ortho- and para-isomer are 5.3×10^{-3} M and 2.85×10^{-3} M, respectively, while the V_{max} values are 3.0×10^{-2} and 6.6×10^{-2} nmol phenol per nmol of cytochrome P-450 per minute, respectively. In other words, the twofold greater enzyme affinity of the para-isomer is paralleled by double the reaction rate.

An example of toxicological relevance is seen in the metabolism of the two isomeric compounds N-2- and N-3-fluorenylacetamide (LVII). While the former is a potent carcinogen, the latter shows only marginal activity. After intraperitoneal (i.p.) administration to rats, biliary excretion of the

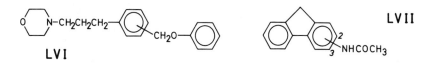

LVI

LVII

TABLE 19
Metabolism of Amphetamine in Rabbit Liver 9000g Supernatant Fractions

		Metabolites			
		1-Phenyl-2-propanol (LV) (mM)		N-Hydroxy-amphetamine (LII) (mM)	
Substrate	Concentration (mM)	1 hr	3 hr	1 hr	3 hr
(R)-Amphetamine	0.90	0.091	0.16	0.093	0.075
(S)-Amphetamine	0.90	0.029	0.098	0.045	0.13
(RS)-Amphetamine	1.80	0.031	0.12	0.049	0.16

		1-Phenyl-2-propanol (LV) (mM)		Phenylacetone oxime (LIII) (mM)	
Substrate	Concentration (mM)	1 hr	3 hr	1 hr	3 hr
(R)-N-Hydroxyamphetamine	0.90	0.002	0.002	0.069	0.20
(S)-N-Hydroxyamphetamine	0.90	0.002	0.002	0.042	0.13

Source: From Ref. 58.

TABLE 20
Stereoselective Formation of Amphetamine Metabolites
in Rabbit Liver 9000g Supernatant Fractions

	R/S ratio (± SD) of metabolites after 1-hr incubation	
	1-Phenyl-2-propanol (LV)	N-Hydroxyamphetamine (LII)
Separate incubations of (R)- and (S)-amphetamine	2.5 ± 0.3	1.4 ± 0.3
Incubations of racemic amphetamine	0.27 ± 0.09	0.20 ± 0.07

Source: From Ref. 59.

N-hydroxylated metabolites accounted for 12.5 ± 4.5% and 0.06 ± 0.03% of
the dose for N-2- and N-3-fluorenylacetamide, respectively [61]. The considerable substrate selectivity of the reaction was confirmed by in vitro studies.
Thus, N-hydroxylation of the 2-isomer by hepatic microsomes of untreated
or 3-methylcholanthrene-treated rats was 40- and 50-fold greater than that
for the 3-isomer. Although this reaction is mediated via cytochrome P-448,
there was no apparent correlation between the magnitude of the binding
spectrum and the extent of N-hydroxylation of the two isomers.

Comparison of the O-demethylation of four regioisomers, namely, 4-,
5-, 6-, and 7-methoxyoxindole (LVIII) [62], by rabbit liver microsomes
showed the extent of demethylation to be in the order of 4 > 5 > 6 > 7 (Table
21). This pattern remains unchanged after phenobarbital pretreatment, although the extent of the reaction is increased twofold (Table 21). Thus, the
stimulation of enzyme activity probably represents quantitative increases
rather than changes in enzyme characteristics. No rationale could be found
to explain the order of demethylation, which was unrelated to the partition
coefficients of the substrates. The observed substrate selectivity may be
due to differences in enzyme affinity as influenced by steric factors, and/or
to topological differences in substrate-enzyme association.

The O-demethylation of the above four methoxyoxindole regioisomers
can be gainfully compared to the N-demethylation of the four stereoisomers
of ephedrine (LIX); see Table 22. The two ephedrine enantiomers have
clearly distinct enzyme affinities, but show identical reaction rates. On the
other hand, the two pseudoephedrine enantiomers exhibit slightly different
values for both K_m and V_{max}. Comparing the four stereoisomers, it appears
that the (1R) and (2S) configurations favor small K_m values, with the influence of the 1-center predominating over that of the 2-center. No conclusions

TABLE 21
O-Demethylation of Methoxyoxindoles (LVIII) by Rabbit Liver Microsomes

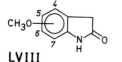

LVIII

	Percentage of demethylation in 1 hr	
	Untreated animals	Phenobarbital-pretreated animals
4-Methoxyoxindole	19	46
5-Methoxyoxindole	14	26
6-Methoxyoxindole	5	11
7-Methoxyoxindole	4	8

Source: From Ref. 62.

can be drawn concerning the V_{max} values since the small differences observed do not reach statistical significance. After 15- and 30-min incubation, however, the isomers with the (2S) configuration have been demethylated at practically the same rate, and at rates 15-25% greater than those of the isomers with the (2R) configuration (Table 22) [63].

In the previous section (III.B), we outlined some of the difficulties encountered in the interpretation of overall metabolic data. For example, some questions concerning the substrate stereoselectivity of para-hydroxy-amphetamine formation were left unanswered. Focusing on individual reactions may be useful, particularly when one is investigating reaction kinetics, as shown in the foregoing few examples. In other cases, however, a clear understanding of reaction kinetics may be difficult to achieve. This is clearly demonstrated in an interesting study of the kinetics of N-demethylation and binding to cytochrome P-450 of three enantiomeric pairs (Table 23) [64]. While there are no significant differences in the K_m values of enantiomers, the V_{max} values differ significantly in two cases. Further, no correlation exists between the kinetics of metabolism and type I binding spectra; in this case, the spectral change is not a visible representation of the Michaelis complex. Little can be drawn from such results with regard to interactions at metabolic sites for these compounds, except that they appear to occur with limited stereoselectivity.

TABLE 22
N-Demethylation of the Ephedrine (LIX) Stereoisomers by Rabbit Liver Preparations

$$\underset{\text{LIX}}{\overset{\displaystyle\bigcirc\!\!-\overset{1}{C}H-\overset{2}{C}H-NHCH_3}{\underset{OHCH_3}{}}}$$

Stereoisomers	K_m ($M \times 10^4$)	V_{max} (nmol HCHO/ mg protein/min)	nmol HCHO/mg protein ($\pm$ SD) after:	
			15 min	30 min
Erythro-isomers				
(1R;2S)-(–)-Ephedrine	1.2	1.3	67.6 ± 1.1	112.4 ± 4.3
(1S;2R)-(+)-Ephedrine	2.7	1.3	54.8 ± 1.1	93.9 ± 2.0
Threo-isomers				
(1R;2R)-(–)-Pseudoephedrine	1.7	1.1	53.7 ± 2.6	88.0 ± 4.2
(1S;2S)-(+)-Pseudoephedrine	2.2	1.8	63.2 ± 2.9	115.3 ± 3.4

Source: From Ref. 63.

TABLE 23
Kinetics of Metabolism and Binding to Cytochrome P-450
of Enantiomeric Substrates in Rat Liver Microsomes

	Metabolism		Binding
Substrate	K_m ($M \times 10^5$)	V_{max}[a]	[spectral dissociation constant K_S ($M \times 10^6$)]
(+)-Propoxyphene	5.44 ± 0.90	75 ± 12[b]	1.21 ± 0.13[b]
(-)-Propoxyphene	5.95 ± 0.95	152 ± 24[b]	0.69 ± 0.13[b]
Dextromethorphan	9.15 ± 0.33	91 ± 12[b]	ND[c]
Levomethorphan	7.71 ± 0.73	144 ± 18[b]	3.53 ± 0.32
(+)-Carbinoxamine	11.34 ± 1.91	117 ± 25	0.68 ± 0.08
(-)-Carbinoxamine	7.95 ± 1.18	89 ± 17	0.68 ± 0.07

[a] V_{max} = nmol HCHO/mg protein/hr.
[b] Statistically significant difference between enantiomers.
[c] Not detectable.
Source: From Ref. 64.

   It would be erroneous, however, to generalize from the preceding example that enantiomeric interactions at metabolic sites show only moderate
stereoselectivity. Consider, for instance, the fate of 5-phenylhydantoin
(LX) in the dog. The yield of urinary (R)-(-)-2-phenylhydantoic acid (LXI)
was approximately 100% of the (R)-form of administered LX; on the other
hand, the absence of (S)-2-phenylhydantoic acid cannot be accounted for
by its further metabolism. A fully stereoselective enzymic attack on

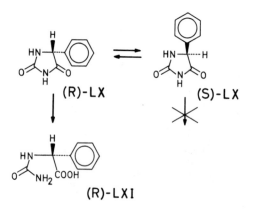

(R)-5-phenylhydantoin would appear to explain these results. But when account was taken of the yield of all metabolites of (R) configuration it became evident that more than 50% of a dose of racemic 5-phenylhydantoin appears in the (R)-form [65].

In order to explain the data it was necessary to propose some process of enantiomeric interconversion. Indeed, the racemization of 5-phenylhydantoin enantiomers has been shown to be catalyzed in neutral pH regions by such species as imidazole, phosphate, and triethanolamine. The in vivo racemization process may thus be either chemically catalyzed or involve a racemase including in its active site an amino, phosphate, or imidazole moiety [66]. Of interest in the present context is the apparently complete stereoselectivity of the enzyme hydrolyzing the hydantoin ring. The same stereoselectivity has been noted in the hydrolysis of 2-phenylsuccinimide (LXII) yielding (R)-(-)-2-phenylsuccinamic acid (LXIII) [67]. Further

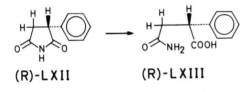

(R)-LXII   **(R)-LXIII**

selectivities of the enzyme are its lack of reactivity toward N-alkylated hydantoins and succinimides, and the fact that it hydrolyzes only the amide bond α, β to the aryl-substituted carbon. Drug-metabolizing enzymes as a rule do not react with apparent total stereoselectivity, as opposed to enzymes acting on endogenous substrates. It is therefore of considerable interest that the aforementioned ring cleavage of 5-phenylhydantoin and 2-phenylsuccinimide results from the action of dihydropyrimidinase (4,5-dihydropyrimidine amidohydrolase), the endogenous substrates of which are dihydrouracil and dihydrothymine [68]. Such an example clearly leads to the conclusion that high or apparently complete substrate selectivity in drug metabolism is a strong indication that endogenous substrate-metabolizing enzymes are involved rather than xenobiotic-metabolizing enzymes. The latter indeed must display low substrate selectivity in order to be operative toward substrates of immense structural variety.

D. Regio- and Stereoselectivity in Conjugation Reactions

The reactivity of ortho- and para-nitrophenol toward rat liver microsomal UDP-glucuronyltransferase differ markedly, the para-isomer being more rapidly conjugated [69]. However, since the substrate concentrations used by Howland and Bohm were not identical (see Table 24), the results cannot be compared in a quantitative manner. This study nevertheless shows the existence of more than one binding site on UDP-glucuronyltransferase.

TABLE 24
Activity of Hepatic Microsomal UDP-glucuronyltransferase
from Adult Rats Toward ortho- and para-Nitrophenol

	Control animals		3-Methylcholanthrene-induced animals	
Substrate	pH	Activity[a]	pH	Activity[a]
ortho-Nitrophenol [b]	5.4[c]	4.1	5.4[c]	15
	7.2[c]	3.0	7.2	10
	9.2[c]	3.8	9.2[c]	34
para-Nitrophenol[b]	5.4[c]	96	5.4[c]	107
	7.2	30	7.2	45
	9.2	36	9.2[c]	62

[a] Activity: nmol product/mg protein/15 min.
[b] Substrate concentration: ortho-isomer 1.0 mM; para-isomer 0.4 mM.
[c] This pH value corresponds to a pH optimum.
Source: From Ref. 69.

Indeed, incubation at different pH values showed three and one pH optima
to exist for activity toward ortho- and para-nitrophenol, respectively,
whereas following pretreatment with 3-methylcholanthrene the enzyme
showed two pH optima toward each substrate. The conjugation of ortho-
nitrophenol at pH 9.2 and 5.4 is inhibited by para-nitrophenol (K_i values ca.
0.1 and 0.06 mM, respectively) and by para-nitrophenyl glucuronide (K_i
values ca. 20.0 and 3.4 mM, respectively), suggesting that at these pH values the two regioisomers bind to the same site. At pH 7.2 on the other hand,
no inhibition of ortho-nitrophenol conjugation was observed, suggesting that
the two substrates do not share the same binding site [69].
    In such studies, regioisomeric substrates are used as a tool to inves-
tigate the properties of a single enzyme (or of multiple forms of a single
enzyme). Regioisomeric compounds may also be substrates for competitive
pathways and thus serve to investigate the relative reactivities of two or
more distinct conjugation pathways. For example, the fate of 1- and 2-
naphthol has been studied in the cat, pig, and rat [70]. The cat is generally
deficient in its ability to form glucuronides of phenols, whereas the pig is
generally deficient in its ability to form sulfate conjugates of phenols; both
pathways are usually readily operative in the rat [71].

TABLE 25
The Conjugation of 1- and 2-Naphthol (25 mg/kg) in the
Cat, Pig, and Rat

Species	1-Naphthol	2-Naphthol
Cat		
^{14}C in 24-hr urine (% dose)	91	73
Percentage of 24-hr excretion present as:		
Glucuronide	1.4	2.6
Sulfate	98	98
Pig		
^{14}C in 24-hr urine (% dose)	81	84
Percentage of 24-hr excretion present as:		
Glucuronide	66	94
Sulfate	32	6
Rat		
^{14}C in 24-hr urine (% dose)	59	86
Percentage of 24-hr excretion present as:		
Glucuronide	47	52
Sulfate	53	48

Source: From Ref. 70.

The data obtained for 1- and 2-naphthol (Table 25) are in agreement
with the species variation just outlined for the cat and the rat. Thus, the
cat excretes almost exclusively 1-naphthyl and 2-naphthyl sulfate from the
corresponding regioisomeric substrate, whereas the rat excretes equal
amounts of glucuronide and sulfate in both cases. But the pig behaves as
expected in the case of 2-naphthol only; quite unexpectedly, significant
amounts of 1-naphthyl sulfate are produced from 1-naphthol. This and other
exceptions, e.g., the significant formation of phenolphthalein glucuronide
in the cat [70], demonstrate that in the conjugation of phenols both species

and substrate influence the relative contribution of the sulfate and glucuronide pathways.

Conjugation reactions may also show substrate stereoselectivity, as
illustrated by propranolol (LXIV). One of the metabolic pathways of this

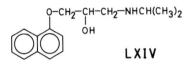

LXIV

chiral drug is the formation of propranolol O-glucuronide; because β-D-
glucuronic acid is optically active, the metabolite exists as two diastereoisomeric forms. However, the relative energies of the two diastereoisomeric metabolites is not expected to influence the substrate stereoselectivity
of the reaction, since this would imply a thermodynamic control. Preliminary studies suggest comparable urinary excretion of (+)- and (-)-pro-
pranolol glucuronide [possibly with a slight excess of the (+)-conjugate (?)]
after administration of the racemate to a patient [72]. In dogs administered
with the separate enantiomers, preferential excretion of the glucuronide of
the (-)-isomer is indicated [72].

The last example to be discussed in this section again involves substrate stereoselectivity, but this time conformational isomerism is considered. Catechol (LXV) and catechol-containing molecules are O-methyl-
ated by catechol-O-methyltransferase (COMT). Recently, benzimidazole
(LXVI) has been shown to be N-methylated by COMT to yield 1-methylbenz-
imidazol (LXVII) [73]. This finding is of interest since it allows some insight into the conformation of catechol when bound to COMT and during
methylation. Indeed, the preferred conformer of catechol is the intra-
molecularly hydrogen-bonded form LXVa; topological analogies between
LXVI and LXVa suggest that the latter conformer of catechol may be the
one recognized and bound by COMT, rather than nonhydrogen-bonded con-
formers such as LXVb.

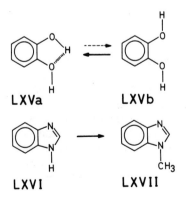

LXVa   LXVb

LXVI   LXVII

IV. PRODUCT REGIOSELECTIVITY

A. The Nature of Product Selectivity

Product selectivity implies that from a given substrate two or more metabolites are generated by competitive pathways at different rates. For example, the oxidation of alcohols occurs competitively with glucuronidation. Thus, in a homologous series of alcohols a decrease in the quantitative importance of the oxidative reactions results in increased glucuronide excretion [72]. In such cases, however, the metabolites are generated by different enzymes and differ widely in their chemical structure. In contrast, the present section and Sec. V will deal with metabolites that are regioisomers or stereoisomers, respectively.

Regioisomeric metabolites may be produced either by the same enzyme* or by two distinct enzymes catalyzing identical reactions. On the other hand, the generation of stereoisomeric metabolites from a single substrate generally implies the involvement of a single enzyme.* In each case, however, the production of regio- and stereoisomeric metabolites results from an enzymic ability to discriminate between two or more closely related sites in the substrate molecule. Regioisomeric metabolites result from the attack of similar groups or atoms differently positioned in the substrate molecule (regiotopic groups), e.g., the ortho, meta, and para positions in a phenyl substituent. The generation of stereoisomeric substrates, as will be discussed in Sec. V, implies an element of prostereoisomerism in the substrate, i.e., diastereotopic or enantiotopic groups.

The enzymic discrimination of regiotopic groups can be explained in various ways. If a substrate binds by a single mode to an enzyme, then the active site of the enzyme must be somewhat flexible in order for it to attack the more reactive or labilized regiotopic site; in such a case, the relative probabilities of the transition states will determine the regioselectivity of the reaction. Alternatively, the substrate may bind to the enzyme by two or more distinct modes, each of which brings one regiotopic group close to the reactive center; in this case, the relative binding energies will determine the regioselectivity, and the various transition states need not have different probabilities.

In short, the hypothesis can be put forward that product regioselectivity is determined either by the different reactivities of regiotopic groups or by steering-group-determined substrate binding. This hypothesis appears to have been verified. Indeed, results given later in this section will indicate a clear preference of monooxygenases for the electron-richer C-H bonds in a given substrate, whereas the highly regio- and stereoselective hydroxylation reactions of steroids by cytochrome P-450 can be explained by the role of steering groups on the substrate molecule which orient the substrate to facilitate attack at specific sites [75].

---

*Which may exist and act in multiple forms.

It can be further postulated that a given substrate may bind to two or more enzymes or enzymic forms catalyzing the same reaction, each of which however acts selectively at alternate regiotopic sites. In this case, the observed regioselectivity will be determined by the relative concentrations of the enzymes, by the relative enzyme-substrate affinity constants, and also by any difference in the transition state energies.

B. Product Regioselectivity in the Hydroxylation of
    Alkyl Groups: Experimental Facts

Alkanes are excellent model compounds for the study of hydroxylating enzymes, and the special attention given to n-alkanes has shown the involvement of several distinct enzyme systems in their metabolism.

The hydroxylation of n-pentane [76] and n-heptane [77] by rat liver microsomes is selective for the $(\omega-1)$-position (Table 26). A careful study of the effects of inducers and inhibitors showed at least three monooxygenases to be active in the hydroxylation of n-heptane, each of these enzymes displaying its own regioselectivity pattern [77]. This and other examples [11] indicate that the regioselectivity observed in the hydroxylation of n-alkanes is determined primarily by the enzymes involved. The properties of the substrate (e.g., molecular size) will have only an indirect effect in "selecting" some enzymes.

Medicinal barbiturates (5-dialkyl-substituted barbituric acids) are also interesting model compounds in the present context. From a review of several studies, it has been concluded that $(\omega-1)$-hydroxylation is preferred for side chains of four or more carbons, whereas 3-carbon chains are hydroxylated more in the (ω)- than $(\omega-1)$-position. Hydroxylation at the $(\omega-2)$-position is documented for some 6-carbon chains [78].

Let us consider the case of amobarbital (LXVIII). Humans receiving the drug do not excrete the unchanged compound in detectable amounts. The major metabolite (50-60% of a dose) is the 3'-hydroxylated derivative (LXIX), in agreement with the rule of $(\omega-1)$-hydroxylation of 4-carbon chains;

TABLE 26
Relative Regioisomeric Hydroxylation of Alkanes by Rat
Liver Microsomes

| Substrate | Position of hydroxylation[a] | | | |
	ω	$\omega-1$	$\omega-2$	$\omega-3$
n-Pentane	<0.5	84	16	--
n-Heptane	9.5	73.8	11.1	5.6

[a] As percentage of total hydroxylation.
Source: Data from Refs. 76 and 77.

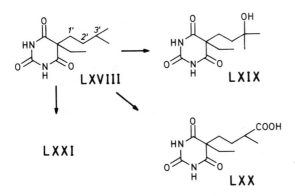

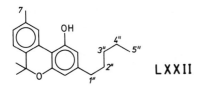

branching at C-3' has no apparent influence on the direction of hydroxylation. A minor metabolite is the carboxylic acid derivative LXX resulting from the rapid oxidation of the (ω)-hydroxylated primary metabolite. An important metabolite (LXXI, ca. 30% of a dose) was believed to be the N-hydroxylated derivative [79] but has now been shown to be N-β-D-glucopyranosylamobarbital [80].

Complex regioselectivity patterns are displayed by molecules containing alkyl chains adjacent to aromatic rings. The ready oxidation of methyl groups adjacent to aromatic rings is common knowledge and is abundantly illustrated in the literature [81]. This phenomenon therefore suggests some activating influence of the aryl group. In the case of ethylbenzene, hydroxylation occurs at the 1'-position (benzylic position) with high regioselectivity [e.g., 82]. But because the hydroxylation of ethylbenzene also occurs with high product stereoselectivity, it will be considered in Sec. V.

In the case of larger alkyl groups adjacent to aromatic rings, preferential benzylic hydroxylation ceases to be the rule—as seen for example with cannabinol [(LXXII); CBN]. Hydroxylation at the 7-position has consistently been found to be the major pathway, while the relative importance

of oxidative attack at the 1"-, 2"-, 3"-, 4"-, and 5"-position varies. The rat is a particularly good hydroxylator, and in this species the 1"- and 4"-positions appear somewhat preferred for hydroxylation over the other sites of the pentyl side chain. The differences in regioselectivity observed between species and between in vivo and in vitro studies indicate that enzymic factors are predominant [83-87].

Valuable confirmation of the mechanistic aspects of benzylic hydroxylation has been obtained by the use of 1,3-diphenylpropane derivatives. These compounds possess three possible sites for aliphatic hydroxylation, namely, two benzylic positions (α and α') and a β-position. As expected, the oxidation of the β-carbon is slight as compared to the attack on the α-carbon and will not be discussed further. On the other hand, the factors influencing the relative hydroxylation of the two benzylic positions are of considerable interest. In the case of 4'-substituted 1,3-diphenylpropane derivatives (LXXIII), it was found that the cytochrome P-450-catalyzed hydroxylation of

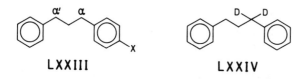

LXXIII   **LXXIV**

the α-position decreased relative to the α'-position with increasing electron-withdrawing capacity of the para-substituent [88]. This means that the less electron density there is in the benzylic position, the less is its reactivity—confirming the electrophilic nature of the biological hydroxylating agent.

When 1,3-diphenylpropane-1,1-d_2 (LXXIV) was used as a substrate for cytochrome P-450-catalyzed hydroxylation, a marked selectivity for the nondeuterated benzylic position was found, as assessed by a significant primary kinetic isotope effect ($k_H/k_D = 11 \pm 1$) [89]. This finding provides fresh evidence that the rate-limiting step in the hydroxylation reaction is the cleavage of a C-H bond.

Regioselective hydroxylation occurs not only in alkyl groups adjacent to aromatic rings but also in alkyl groups adjacent to isolated double or triple bonds. In the case of carbon-carbon double bonds, there are many examples of the preferred oxidation of the α-carbon (allylic position). For example, 5-cycloalkenyl-substituted barbiturates are selectively hydroxylated at the allylic position(s), as recently reviewed [11]. Another interesting example is provided by the biotransformation of methylcyclohexene (LXXV) in rabbits. Two alcohols were recovered from the urine; the major and minor metabolites were the 3- and 6-hydroxylated derivatives, respectively [90]. The oxidative attack in this instance occurred only at the allylic positions, with the less sterically hindered position being preferred.

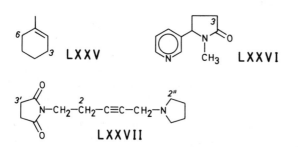

Other groups rendering the α-carbon open to attack include the amide group and the carbon-carbon triple bond. An example of regioselectivity alpha to an amide grouping is seen in the 3-hydroxylation of cotinine (LXXVI), a metabolite of nicotine [91]. Hydroxylation alpha to an acetylenic bond also has been discovered recently in the metabolism of N-(5-pyrrolidino-3-pentynyl)succinimide (LXXVII); the biotransformation of this compound by rat liver 9000g supernatant yields the metabolites hydroxylated at carbon-3' (alpha to an amide group), at carbon-2" (alpha to an amino group, as will be discussed next), and the α-acetylenic alcohol (hydroxylation at C-2) [92].

The most frequently encountered examples of regioselective hydroxylation occur at carbon atoms alpha to heteroatoms such as nitrogen and oxygen. Such hydroxylations are the initial step in N- and O-dealkylation pathways; their marked predominance as compared to their regiotopic sites (C_β, C_γ, ...) is common knowledge and has been extensively discussed [e.g., 11]. To illustrate this type of regioselectivity, let us consider N-n-propylamphetamine (LXXVIII), the metabolism of which has been investigated

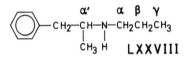

in rat liver homogenates [93]. Metabolites resulting from α'-hydroxylation followed by deamination account for 3-7% of all metabolites, while the N-oxidized metabolites account for some 20-40%. On the other hand, metabolites resulting from C_α- and C_β-hydroxylation represent 35-40% and 3-6% of all metabolites, respectively. In this instance, therefore, there is a 10-fold predominance of C_α- over C_β-hydroxylation.

Phenacetin (LXXIX) undergoes O-dealkylation as the major biotransformation route. A comparatively weak C_β-hydroxylation has also been characterized, yielding metabolites LXXXI and LXXXIII [94; cf. references therein].

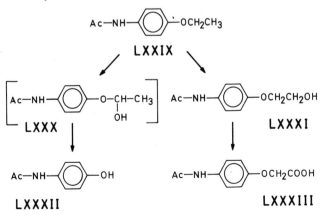

The foregoing examples suggest that the electronic influence of the heteroatom determines the observed C_α-regioselectivity. This hypothesis has been confirmed by theoretical studies presented in Sec. IV.C. However, such electronic factors are not alone in influencing the hydroxylation of alkyl groups adjacent to heteroatoms. Enzymic factors can sometimes be characterized, as shown in the oxidation of propyl para-nitrophenyl ether by rat liver preparations. Indeed, while C_β-hydroxylation is seen with normal animals, O-dealkylation predominates following phenobarbital induction [95].

The demethylation of sterically nonequivalent N-methyl or O-methyl groups can also be fruitfully discussed within the context of product regioselectivity. Quite often the chemical and physicochemical properties of such groups differ very little, and minute external influences may suffice in determining regioselectivity.

Papaverine (LXXXIV) contains four methoxy groups showing metabolic nonequivalence [96]. Thus, while no 3'-O-demethylation was found to occur, marked species variation was detected in the biliary excretion of other O-demethylated metabolites (Table 27). It appears that 4'-O-demethylation is

TABLE 27
Regioselective O-Demethylation of Papaverine
(LXXXIV) in Various Species

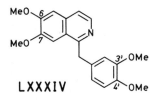

Species	Mean percent of dose in 6-hr bile	Metabolites in the bile[a]			
		4'-OH	7-OH	6-OH	4',6-(OH)$_2$
Rat	84	42	35	10	3
Guinea pig	50	53	29	11	2
Rabbit	44	53	7	33	2
Dog	57	68	4	14	7
Cat	50	17	4	62	5

[a] As percentage of total radioactivity chromatographed.
Source: From Ref. 96.

TABLE 28
Regioselective N-Demethylation of Caffeine (LXXXV) in the Rat

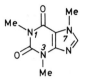

LXXXV

	Site		
	N-1	N-7	N-3
Total urinary excretion of metabolites being demethylated at specified site[a]	12%	20%	25%
pK_a of dimethylxanthine isomer having unsubstituted specified site	9.9	8.7	8.5

[a] In percentage of dose.
Source: From Ref. 98.

a major route in all species except the cat. On the other hand, 7-O-de-methylation is an important route in the rat and guinea pig only, and 6-O-demethylation is significant in the rabbit and the major route in the cat. These species variations can be explained in terms of differences in enzymic activities or by the presence of several enzymes in varying proportions.

Another relevant example is provided by caffeine (LXXXV); older metabolic studies have been criticized [97], but a recent and extensive study has provided a good understanding of its metabolism in the rat [98]. Summation of all metabolites demethylated at positions 1, 7, and 3 shows the relative amount to increase in that order (Table 28). Comparison of the amount of N-1-, N-7-, and N-3-demethylated metabolites with the pK_a values of the dimethylxanthine isomers having a hydrogen atom at positions 1, 7, or 3 (theobromine, theophylline, and paraxanthine, respectively) shows the acidity at each site to increase with the calculated percentage of demethylation. Such a trend indicates electronic factors to be operative in determining regioselectivity, although the nature of these factors remains unknown.

TABLE 49
Substituent Parameters Used in the QSAR Study of N-Diethylglycinanilides

Substituent	f^a	V^b	$\underline{F}^c$	$\underline{R}^c$
H	0.20	2.5	0.00	0.00
Methoxy	0.25	16.87	0.26	-0.51
n-Propoxy	1.30	37.33	0.22	-0.45
n-Butoxy	1.83	47.56	0.25	-0.55
n-Pentyloxy	2.36	57.79	0.25	-0.57
n-Hexyloxy	2.88	68.02	0.25	-0.57
n-Octyloxy	3.94	88.48	0.25	-0.57

[a] Hydrophobic fragmental constant according to Rekker [17].
[b] Group volume in cm^3/mol [189].
[c] Data from Hansch et al. [204].

a statistically sound equation [(Eq. (19)] may be misleading in a physical sense.

$$\log RRH = -0.204(\pm 0.032)\, f_{ortho} - 0.285(\pm 0.032)\, f_{meta}$$
$$-0.416(\pm 0.032)\, f_{para} + 1.45(\pm 0.07) \tag{16}$$
$$n = 19;\ r^2 = 0.922;\ s = 0.134;\ F = 59.1$$

$$\log RRH = -0.0104(\pm 0.0015)\, V_{ortho} - 0.0138(\pm 0.0015)\, V_{meta}$$
$$-0.0195(\pm 0.0015)\, V_{para} + 1.53(\pm 0.08) \tag{17}$$
$$n = 19;\ r^2 = 0.921;\ s = 0.135;\ F = 58.6$$

$$\log RRH = -0.302(\pm 0.045)\, f_{subt} + 1.33(\pm 0.10) \tag{18}$$
$$n = 19;\ r^2 = 0.727;\ s = 0.237;\ F = 45.2$$

$$\log RRH = -0.287(\pm 0.026)\, f_{subt} + 0.00347(\pm 0.00120)\, V_{ortho}$$
$$-0.00558(\pm 0.00120)\, V_{para} + 1.34(\pm 0.05) \tag{19}$$
$$n = 19;\ r^2 = 0.944;\ s = 0.115;\ F = 83.6$$

$$\log RRH = -0.299(\pm 0.017)\, f_{subt} + 0.828(\pm 0.199)\, \underline{F}_{ortho}$$
$$-1.30(\pm 0.20)\, \underline{F}_{para} + 1.36(\pm 0.04) \tag{20}$$
$$n = 19;\ r^2 = 0.967;\ s = 0.088;\ F = 145$$

$$\log RRH = -0.297(\pm 0.017)\ f_{subt} - 0.371(\pm 0.091)\ \underline{R}_{ortho}$$
$$+ 0.603(\pm 0.091)\ \underline{R}_{para} + 1.36(\pm 0.04) \tag{21}$$
$$n = 19;\ r^2 = 0.967;\ s = 0.087;\ F = 148$$

$$\log RRH = -0.295(\pm 0.016)\ f_{subt} + 0.819(\pm 0.194)\ \underline{F}_{ortho}$$
$$+ 0.602(\pm 0.089)\ \underline{R}_{para} + 1.35(\pm 0.04) \tag{22}$$
$$n = 19;\ r^2 = 0.968;\ s = 0.086;\ F = 154$$

$$\log RRH = -0.311(\pm 0.016)\ f_{subt} + 0.378(\pm 0.093)\ I_{ortho}$$
$$+ 0.197(\pm 0.093)\ I_{meta} - 0.145(\pm 0.093)\ I_{para} + 1.21(\pm 0.08)$$
$$n = 19;\ r^2 = 0.974;\ s = 0.081;\ F = 129 \tag{23}$$

Examining f_{subt} together with electronic parameters yields Eqs. (20) to (22), which explore the influences of inductive and mesomeric effects with increased significance as compared to the V parameters (the meta terms are nonsignificant). An inductive electron withdrawal at the ortho position increases the rate of hydrolysis, while the reverse holds for the para position. The mesomeric parameters show opposite effects.

Equations (20) to (22) may appear as highly satisfactory. However, Table 49 shows no spread at all in the values of $\underline{F}$ and $\underline{R}$; there is no exploration of electronic spaces, and Eqs. (20) to (22) must be considered with care. In fact, the input values of $\underline{F}$ and $\underline{R}$ are so close that they behave like indicator variables. In Eq. (23), they have been effectively replaced by three indicator variables (I) which take the value of 1 or 0 depending on whether the particular position is substituted or not. Equation (23) is the "best" equation: highest r^2 and F, smallest s. This equation indicates that, when the lipophilic effect is adequately accounted for, the rate of hydrolysis is increased by the occupation of the ortho and meta position and decreased by the occupation of the para position. No supposition is made in Eq. (23) as to which effect or combination of effects (electronic, etc.) influence log RRH, because the molecules investigated allow no such hypothesis to be verified.

E. Inhibition of the para-Hydroxylation of Aniline by Alcohols

Aniline, a type II compound, is para-hydroxylated by rat liver microsomes, and the reaction is inhibited by ethanol. Cohen and Mannering [206] have reported the inhibitory activities of 22 alcohols (linear, branched, and one aromatic). They have also shown that a parabolic relationship exists between the log of I_{50} and log P.

The alcohols, with their log P and log $1/I_{50}$ values, are listed in Table 50. A general and schematic representation of the aliphatic alcohols investigated is given in diagram CLXIX. In order to test the influence of molecular steric properties on I_{50}, we have used as input parameters the

TABLE 50
Inhibition of the Microsomal para-Hydroxylation of Aniline by Alcohols

Alcohol	log P[a]	log 1/I_{50}[b] exp.	log 1/I_{50}[b] calc.[c]
Methanol	-0.66	-3.09	-2.62
Ethanol	-0.32	-1.10	-1.59
n-Propanol	0.34	-0.48	-0.59
n-Butanol	0.88	-0.05	0.04
n-Pentanol	1.40	0.27	0.17
n-Hexanol	1.84	0.54	0.83
n-Heptanol	2.34	0.68	0.16
2-Propanol	0.14	-0.47	-0.51
1-Methylpropanol	0.61	-0.35	-0.21
1-Methylbutanol	1.14	-0.07	0.16
1-Methylpentanol	1.64	0.15	0.08
1-Methylhexanol	2.14	0.25	0.48
3-Pentanol	1.14	-0.37	-0.27
2-Methyl-3-pentanol	1.41	-0.89	-0.70
2,4-Dimethyl-3-pentanol	1.71	-1.38	-1.26
2-Methylbutanol	1.14	-0.15	-0.27
3-Methylbutanol	1.14	-0.19	0.16
Neopentanol	1.36	-0.67	-0.69
tert-Pentanol	0.89	-2.56	0.04[d]
3-Hexanol	1.61	-0.47	-0.33
2-Methylpropanol	0.61	-0.39	-0.65
Benzyl alcohol	1.10	0.32	-0.28

[a] Data from Hansch et al. [207] and Leo et al. [208].
[b] I_{50} = inhibitory concentration (in mM) required for a 50% reduction in enzyme activity.
[c] Calculated according to Eq. (27).
[d] Not included in the derivation of Eqs. (24) to (27).
Source: From Ref. 206.

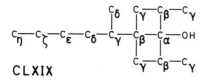

CLXIX

number of carbon atoms in the β, γ, δ, ϵ, and ζ positions. In the stepwise procedure of the multiple linear regression analysis, the first variable entered is log P, followed by (number C_γ) to give Eq. (24), which is statistically poor. The third variable to enter is $(\log P)^2$, yielding the much improved Eq. (25). The latter clearly indicates a parabolic relationship between $\log 1/I_{50}$ and log P. It must be noted, however, that tert-pentanol is an outlier in these equations, for steric and/or electronic reasons, and it has been removed from the calculations. We have investigated whether the addition of a further variable to Eq. (25) was statistically permissible; this was the case for (number C_ϵ) and (number C_ζ), yielding Eqs. (26) and (27).

$$\log 1/I_{50} = 0.925(\pm 0.185) \log P - 0.335(\pm 0.136) \text{ (number } C_\gamma)$$
$$- 0.897 \ (\pm 0.235) \tag{24}$$
$$n = 21; \ r^2 = 0.582; \ s = 0.551; \ F = 12.5$$

$$\log 1/I_{50} = - 0.633(\pm 0.123) \ (\log P)^2 + 2.14(\pm 0.26) \log P$$
$$- 0.544(\pm 0.097) \text{ (number } C_\gamma) - 0.827(\pm 0.152) \tag{25}$$
$$n = 21; \ r^2 = 0.836; \ s = 0.355; \ F = 28.9$$

$$\log 1/I_{50} = - 0.681(\pm 0.118) \ (\log P)^2 + 2.00(\pm 0.26) \log P$$
$$- 0.444(\pm 0.105) \text{ (number } C_\gamma)$$
$$+ 0.458(\pm 0.249) \text{ (number } C_\epsilon) - 0.866(\pm 0.144) \tag{26}$$
$$n = 21; \ r^2 = 0.865; \ s = 0.332; \ F = 25.6$$
$$t \text{ for (number } C_\epsilon) = 1.84 \ (\alpha = 0.08)$$

$$\log 1/I_{50} = - 0.847(\pm 0.146) \ (\log P)^2 + 2.19(\pm 0.239) \log P$$
$$- 0.435(\pm 0.099) \text{ (number } C_\gamma)$$
$$+ 0.904(\pm 0.401) \text{ (number } C_\zeta) - 0.803(\pm 0.137) \tag{27}$$
$$n = 21; \ r^2 = 0.876; \ s = 0.319; \ F = 28.2$$
$$t \text{ for (number } C_\zeta) = 2.25 \ (\alpha = 0.04)$$

A t-test analysis shows a better significance for the latter than for the former variable. The "best" equation is thus Eq. (27); it indicates an optimal log P value of 1.30 and shows that the inhibitory power is decreased by increasing the number of γ carbons. The latter relationship can be understood as meaning that, at a distance from the OH group corresponding to γ carbons, too much steric crowding decreases the affinity to the binding site. On the other hand, lengthening the chain to populate positions ϵ and ζ considerably increases the affinity for the alcohol-binding site. Equation (27), however, shows a good but not excellent correlation coefficient, and other parameters, presumably electronic, may be needed to improve the correlation and incorporate tert-pentanol.

F. Interaction of Hydrocarbons with Cytochrome P-450

Tichý [209] has reported the spectral dissociation constant of the complexes formed between rat liver microsomal cytochrome P-450 and hydrocarbons inducing type I difference spectra. A total of 29 compounds were investigated (Table 51), comprising arenes, alkanes, cycloalkanes, cycloalkenes, and arylalkanes.

Equations (28) and (29) show that $\log 1/(\text{rel } K_S)$ is poorly correlated with $\log P$, linearly as well as parabolically. The hypothesis has therefore been formulated that structural factors play a significant role in the complex stability, and particularly that the saturated and unsaturated moieties should contribute differently. To test this hypothesis, we have used as variables V_{ali}, the volume of the saturated moiety in a given substrate (comprising all sp^3 carbons and adjacent hydrogens), and V_π, the volume of the unsaturated moiety (comprising all sp^2 carbons and adjacent hydrogens). Taken independently V_π and V_{ali} do not correlate with $\log 1/(\text{rel } K_S)$, the r^2 terms being 0.098 and 0.035, respectively. However, taken together

TABLE 51
Relative Spectral Dissociation Constant for the Interaction of
Hydrocarbons with Cytochrome P-450

Substrate	$\log P^a$	V_π^b	V_{ali}^b	$\log 1/(\text{rel } K_S)^c$	
				exp.	calc.[d]
Benzene	2.13	48.36	0.	-0.939	-0.353
Naphthalene	3.37	73.97	0.	0.723	0.469
Anthracene	4.45	99.58	0.	1.445	1.291
Phenanthrene	4.46	99.58	0.	1.310	1.291
Pyrene	5.44	109.04	0.	1.310	1.594
Diphenyl	4.04	91.68	0.	1.207	1.037
Acenaphthene	4.13	68.93	20.46	1.039	0.925

TABLE 51 (continued)

Substrate	log P[a]	V_π[b]	V_{ali}[b]	log $1/(rel\ K_S)$[c] exp.	calc.[d]
Fluorene	4.30	87.64	10.23	1.282	1.216
Toluene	2.60	45.84	13.67	-0.230	-0.021
ortho-Xylene	3.12	43.32	27.34	0.164	0.311
meta-Xylene	3.20	43.32	27.34	0.282	0.311
para-Xylene	3.15	43.32	27.34	0.071	0.311
para-Cymene	4.06	43.32	47.79	0.611	0.929
Dibenzyl	4.85	91.68	20.46	1.641	1.655
Diphenylmethane	4.03	91.68	10.23	1.407	1.346
n-Hexane	4.00	0.	68.26	-0.137	0.157
n-Heptane	4.58	0.	78.49	0.372	0.466
n-Octane	5.16	0.	88.72	0.527	0.775
Cyclohexane	3.48	0.	61.38	0.000	0.051
Cycloheptane	4.06	0.	71.61	0.164	0.258
Cyclooctane	4.64	0.	81.84	0.942	0.567
Decaline	5.28	0.	95.40	1.403	0.977
Perhydroanthracene	7.08	0.	129.42	2.039	2.004
Perhydrophenanthrene	7.08	0.	129.42	1.762	2.004
Methylcyclohexane	4.06	0.	71.60	0.346	0.258
Cyclohexene	2.99	16.94	40.92	0.393	-0.125
Cyclohexadiene	2.49	33.88	20.46	0.039	-0.199
Cyclooctatetraene	2.66	67.76	0.	0.445	0.270
Tetraline	3.83	43.32	40.92	0.778	0.721

[a] Calculated according to Rekker [17].
[b] Values in cm^3/mol calculated according to Bondi [189].
[c] rel K_S = relative spectral dissociation constant (cyclohexane = 1.00).
[d] Calculated from Eq. (30).
Source: From Ref. 209.

the two parameters explain 87% of the variance in the dependent variable: Eq. (30) indicates that a good correlation has been achieved. It shows also that the affinity for the enzyme in the complex increases with molecular size (the coefficients of V_π and V_{ali} have positive signs) and that the unsaturated region contributes somewhat more to the affinity than does the saturated region.

$$\log 1/(\text{rel } K_s) = 0.466(\pm 0.070) \log P - 1.20(\pm 0.30) \tag{28}$$

$$n = 29; \; r^2 = 0.623; \; s = 0.436; \; F = 44.7$$

$$\log 1/(\text{rel } K_s) = -0.0512(\pm 0.0400) (\log P)^2 + 0.931(\pm 0.371) \log P$$

$$- 2.18(\pm 0.82) \tag{29}$$

$$n = 29; \; r^2 = 0.645; \; s = 0.431; \; F = 23.7$$

$$\log 1/(\text{rel } K_s) = 0.0321(\pm 0.0024) V_\pi + 0.0302(\pm 0.0024) V_{ali} - 1.90(\pm 0.20)$$

$$n = 29; \; r^2 = 0.875; \; s = 0.256; \; F = 90.9 \tag{30}$$

$$\log P = 0.0429(\pm 0.0008) V_\pi + 0.0553(\pm 0.0008) V_{ali} \tag{31}$$

$$n = 29; \; r^2 = 0.997; \; s = 0.251; \; F = 4160$$

Equation (31) shows another interesting fact, namely, that V_π and V_{ali} together are almost perfectly correlated with log P. This indicates the compatibility and reciprocal consistency of two independent sets of parameters: the hydrophobic fragmental constant [17] and the group volumes [189]. From Eq. (31) it can be seen that for equal volumes the saturated moiety contributes more to the log P of a hydrocarbon than does the unsaturated moiety. Note that Eq. (31) has no constant, for the physical interpretation of such a constant would be difficult or impossible. Preliminary studies generated an equation ($r^2 = 0.957$) including a constant term, the null hypothesis of which had a probability of 81%; Eq. (31) was therefore forced through the origin using a built-in option of the statistical program.

G. Metabolic Parameters of Barbiturates

Some homologous series of barbiturates (CLXX) have recently been examined for their spectral dissociation constant with rat liver microsomal cytochrome P-450 and for their hepatic clearance using the isolated perfused rat liver [210]. The compounds investigated and their physicochemical parameters are listed in Table 52, while Table 53 gives the metabolic responses. It must be noted that the substituent R_3 is not considered by means of its volume, as is the case for R_1 and R_2, but by the indicator variable I. Indeed, R_3 is either H or CH_3; any pair of numbers would be suitable parameters, hence the simplest set, 0 and 1.

TABLE 52
Physicochemical Parameters of Barbiturates (CLXX)

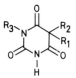

CLXX

Barbiturate	f_{subt}[a]	V_1[b]	V_2[c]	I[d]
1. Propylethylbarbituric acid	3.46	23.9	34.13	0
2. Butylethyl-	3.98	23.9	44.36	0
3. Pentylethyl-	4.51	23.9	54.59	0
4. Isopentylethyl-	4.39	23.9	54.58	0
5. s-Pentylethyl-	4.39	23.9	54.58	0
6. (2,3-Dimethylbutyl)ethyl-	4.81	23.9	64.8	0
7. Hexylethyl-	5.04	23.9	64.82	0
8. Heptylethyl-	5.56	23.9	75.05	0
9. Octylethyl-	6.09	23.9	85.28	0
10. Nonylethyl-	6.62	23.9	95.51	0
11. Aprobarbital	3.57	30.64	34.12	0
12. Talbutal	4.10	30.64	44.35	0
13. Nealbarbital	4.71	30.64	54.57	0
14. Secobarbital	4.62	30.64	54.58	0
15. Brallobarbital	3.54	30.64	40.77	0
16. Bromoallylisopropyl-	3.72	34.12	40.77	0
17. Butallylonal	4.25	40.77	44.35	0
18. Bromoallyl-(1-methylbutyl)-	4.77	40.77	54.58	0
19. N-Methylbrallobarbital	3.77	30.64	40.77	1
20. Narcobarbital	3.95	34.12	40.77	1
21. N-Methylbutallylonal	4.48	40.77	44.35	1
22. Norhexobarbital	3.75	13.67	53.27	0

TABLE 52 (continued)

Barbiturate	f_{subt} [a]	V_1 [b]	V_2 [c]	I [d]
23. Cyclopentobarbital	3.95	30.64	43.04	0
24. Cyclobarbital	4.28	23.9	53.27	0
25. Heptabarbital	4.81	23.9	63.5	0
26. Reposal[R]	4.76	23.9	66.43	0
27. Hexobarbital	3.98	13.67	53.27	1
28. N-Methylcyclopentobarbital	4.18	30.64	43.04	1
29. N-Methylcyclobarbital	4.51	23.9	53.27	1
30. N-Methylphenobarbital	3.83	23.9	45.84	1
31. N-Methylheptabarbital	5.04	23.9	63.5	1
32. N-Methylreposal	4.99	23.9	66.43	1

[a] Sum of fragmental constants [17] of substituents R_1, R_2, and R_3.
[b] Volume in cm^3/mol [189] of R_1.
[c] Volume of R_2, the larger C-5 substituent.
[d] I = 0 when R_3 = H; I = 1 when R_3 = methyl.

Investigation of the spectral dissociation constant showed $\log 1/K_S$ to be strongly dependent upon the overall lipophilicity of substituents, and upon the bulk of the individual substituents. However, the correlation is satisfactory only upon addition of a squared term, either f_{subt}^2 or V_2^2; the high cross-correlation of the two terms forbids their use in the same equation.

Equation (32) indicates that the affinity for the enzyme increases up to an optimal f_{subt} value of 4.65, and then decreases. Replacing f_{subt}^2 by V_2^2 to yield Eq. (33) renders f_{subt} nonsignificant and forces its exclusion. Equation (33) is interesting in that it shows how the largest substituent (R_2) controls the affinity, which is found to increase up to an optimal V_2 value of 73.6 cm^3/mol (i.e., very close to the volume of a n-heptyl group; see compound 8 in Table 52), and decreases for the n-octyl and n-nonyl substituents.

In Eqs. (32) and (33), V_1 and I have positive coefficients of comparable value, indicating that they contribute positively to the affinity. Equation (32) gives a positive coefficient for V_2; this sign is misleading physically since we know from Eq. (33) that the relationship of $\log 1/K_S$ with V_2 is that of a parabola with a maximum.

The QSAR of the relative hepatic clearance (RHC) are explored in Eqs. (34) to (36). The two parameters contributing the most to this biological response are I, as an index of substitution at N-1, and f_{subt}, with which a

TABLE 53
Metabolic Parameters of Barbiturates in the Rat

Barbiturate[a]	log $1/K_s$[b]		log RHC[d]	
	exp.	calc.[c]	exp.	calc.[e]
1	0.63	0.55	-2.40	-2.06
2	1.05	1.05	-1.17	-1.28
3	1.49	1.40	-0.54	-0.67
4	1.42	1.39	-0.79	-0.66
5	1.35	1.39	-0.51	-0.66
6	1.60	1.63	-0.37	-0.15
7	1.72	1.60	-0.09	-0.23
8	1.70	1.65	0.01	0.05
9	1.62	1.55	0.05	0.14
10	1.25	1.29	0.21	0.06
11	0.66	0.74	-1.82	-1.81
12	1.01	1.21	-1.18	-1.06
13	1.21	1.53	-1.31	-0.50
14	1.55	1.53	-0.52	-0.48
15	0.87	0.87	-1.43	-1.44
16	0.98	1.03	-1.33	-1.26
17	1.51	1.43	-0.50	-0.74
18	1.89	1.71	-0.02	-0.21
19	0.99	1.31	-0.57	-0.60
20	1.47	1.45	-0.28	-0.45
21	1.92	1.78	-0.23	0.01
22	1.00	0.97	-1.04	-1.14
23	1.10	1.13	-0.87	-1.16
24	1.39	1.34	-0.52	-0.73
25	1.66	1.60	0.00	-0.22
26	1.59	1.67	-0.12	-0.04

TABLE 53 (continued)

| Barbiturate | $\log 1/K_s$[b] | | $\log RHC$[d] | |
	exp.	calc.[c]	exp.	calc.[e]
27	1.44	1.38	-0.09	-0.33
28	1.60	1.51	0.10	-0.38
29	1.62	1.68	0.19	0.00
30	1.64	1.33	-1.12	-0.49
31	1.82	1.88	0.41	0.44
32	1.77	1.96	0.39	0.63

[a] Numbers represent barbiturates listed in Table 52.
[b] K_s = spectral dissociation constant in mM.
[c] Calculated from Eq. (32).
[d] RHC = relative hepatic clearance (heptabarbital = 1.00).
[e] Calculated from Eq. (35).
Source: From Ref. 210.

parabolic relationship exists, suggesting that the hepatic clearance is governed mainly (81% of the variance) by the overall lipophilicity of the molecule and by the presence or absence of a methyl group at N-1. Indeed, the
presence of the latter considerably increases the metabolic clearance, suggesting the methyl group to be a preferred site of enzymic attack.

$$\log 1/K_s = -0.274(\pm 0.035)\, f_{subt}^2 + 2.55(\pm 0.37)\, f_{subt}$$
$$+ 0.0179(\pm 0.0072)\, V_1 + 0.0228(\pm 0.0106)\, V_2$$
$$+ 0.310\,(\pm 0.059)\, I - 6.20(\pm 0.80) \tag{32}$$
$$n = 32;\ r^2 = 0.862;\ s = 0.141;\ F = 32.4;\ f_o = 4.65$$

$$\log 1/K_s = 0.0249(\pm 0.0043)\, V_1 - 0.000740(\pm 0.000095)\, V_2^2$$
$$+ 0.109(\pm 0.012)\, V_2 + 0.328(\pm 0.057)\, I - 2.98(\pm 0.41) \tag{33}$$
$$n = 32;\ r^2 = 0.856;\ s = 0.141;\ F = 40.2;\ V_{2/o} = 73.6$$

$$\log RHC = -0.290(\pm 0.076)\, f_{subt}^2 + 3.51(\pm 0.74)\, f_{subt}$$
$$+ 0.655(\pm 0.124)\, I - 10.5(\pm 1.8) \tag{34}$$
$$n = 32;\ r^2 = 0.806;\ s = 0.310;\ F = 38.9;\ f_o = 6.05$$

$$\log \text{RHC} = -0.309(\pm 0.070) \; f_{\text{subt}}^2 + 2.67(\pm 0.75) \; f_{\text{subt}}$$
$$+ \; 0.0300(\pm 0.0146) \; V_1 + 0.0576(\pm 0.0215) \; V_2$$
$$+ \; 0.743(\pm 0.119) \; I - 10.3(\pm 1.6) \tag{35}$$
$$n = 32; \; r^2 = 0.849; \; s = 0.285; \; F = 29.2; \; f_o = 4.32$$

$$\log \text{RHC} = 0.0312(\pm 0.0089) \; V_1 - 0.000811(\pm 000195) \; V_2^2$$
$$+ \; 0.748(\pm 0.115) \; I - 6.68(\pm 0.84) + 0.141(\pm 0.024) \; V_2 \tag{36}$$
$$n = 32; \; r^2 = 0.839; \; s = 0.288; \; F = 35.2; \; V_{2/o} = 86.9$$

The addition of V_1 and V_2 (statistically significant in the Student's t-test) in Eq. (34) results in Eq. (35), which displays somewhat better statistics. Interestingly, the optimal value of f_{subt} (f_o) varies markedly when going from one equation to the other; in Eq. (35), f_o is comparable to that in Eq. (32). This variation indicates that Eq. (34), despite its level of significance, displaces on the f_{subt} and I terms the contributions of V_1 and V_2, thereby somewhat distorting their regression coefficients. As was the case with $\log 1/K_s$ [Eq. (33)], the dependent variable $\log$ RHC can also be expressed as a parabolic function of V_2 (but not of V_1), resulting in Eq. (36) from which the f_{subt} term is excluded. The maximum hepatic clearance is predicted for a n-octyl substituent at C-5.

The relationship between the hepatic clearance and the binding constant is examined in Eqs. (37) and (38). It can be seen that together with an increased affinity for cytochrome P-450 there is a corresponding increase in hepatic elimination [Eq. (37)]; R_2 and R_3 also play a positive role [Eq. (38)], presumably by increasing the metabolic disposition of the compounds.

$$\log \text{RHC} = 1.61(\pm 0.19) \; \log 1/K_s - 2.78(\pm 0.28) \tag{37}$$
$$n = 32; \; r^2 = 0.696; \; s = 0.375; \; F = 68.8$$

$$\log \text{RHC} = 0.981(\pm 0.197) \; \log 1/K_s + 0.0219(\pm 0.0047) \; V_2$$
$$+ \; 0.425(\pm 0.133) \; I - 3.21(\pm 0.24) \tag{38}$$
$$n = 32; \; r^2 = 0.836; \; s = 0.286; \; F = 47.5$$

H. Pharmacokinetics of N-Alkylated Amphetamines in Humans

Our final example will be devoted to the in vivo metabolism and disposition of amphetamines in humans. Suitable quantitative data are rare because they require two distinct and consecutive studies, namely, a metabolic study generating data such as percentages of metabolism and concentration of metabolites, followed by a pharmacokinetic investigation to calculate rate constants. The latter provide the most meaningful biological responses for QSAR studies. We were therefore pleased to find an extensive study [211] reporting the metabolism of amphetamine and 14 N-alkyl derivatives (CLXXI) in three volunteers, and analyzing the results in terms of an elaborate multiple compartment model. The biological data in Table 54 are the mean values for the three volunteers as published by Donike and collaborators [211]. Our QSAR study yields good to very good correlations—unexpectedly good considering that only two out of the three subjects had controlled acidic urine to minimize tubular reasorption of basic metabolites.

The parameters used in the study are log P, the number of hydrogen atoms on C_α of the N-alkyl group as an index of steric accessibility of C_α to monooxygenation, and pK_a values.

Equations (39) to (40) show that log PCU (log of the percentage of drug being excreted unchanged) is parabolically related to log P with a high degree of statistical significance. Benzylamphetamine is an outlier in these equations and has not been included in the calculations; it is excreted too slowly and in too small an amount as compared to the predictions of Eqs. (39) and (40). Its decreased basicity as compared to N-alkylamphetamines should result in an increased tubular reabsorption explaining this discrepancy. Indeed, an equation has been derived including both log P and pK_a [Eq. (41)], in which benzylamphetamine is no more an outlier. This equation, from which a square term and the constant had to be rejected, has only a marginal interest because all pK_a values except one (benzylamphetamine) are almost identical.

$$\log PCU = - 0.725(\pm 0.081) \log P + 3.61(\pm 0.29) \tag{39}$$

$$n = 14; \ r^2 = 0.870; \ s = 0.294; \ F = 80.4$$

$$\log PCU = - 0.164(\pm 0.041) (\log P)^2 + 0.521(\pm 0.321) \log P + 1.41(\pm 0.59) \tag{40}$$

$$n = 14; \ r^2 = 0.946; \ s = 0.198; \ F = 96.5; \ \log P_0 = 1.59$$

$$\log PCU = - 0.721(\pm 0.075) \log P + 0.361(\pm 0.028) pK_a \tag{41}$$

$$n = 15; \ r^2 = 0.954; \ s = 0.294; \ F = 136$$

As regards the rate constant of renal excretion, the only sound equation we have been able to derive is Eq. (42), which shows quantitatively how an increased lipophilicity decreases the renal excretion, a phenomenon obviously related to tubular reabsorption. The inclusion of any other parameter was not significant, and benzylamphetamine is an outlier in this equation.

The pharmacokinetic investigations of Donike and collaborators [211] allowed them to calculate the rate constant of the first dealkylation. For this biological response, 17 observations are at hand since three compounds are N-methyl-N-alkyl derivatives undergoing two distinct reactions of first dealkylation. Log k_1 shows a linear, positive correlation with log P [Eq. (43)]; the correlation is not improved by a squared term. On the other hand, the introduction of the additional parameter (number of H atoms on C_α) yields an interesting and statistically fair equation [Eq. (44)]. This

TABLE 54
Pharmacokinetics of N-Alkylated Amphetamines in Humans (CLXXI)

CLXXI

Amphetamine derivative	log P[a]	pK$_a$[b]	log PCU[c] exp.	log PCU[c] calc.[d]	log EXC[e] exp.	log EXC[e] calc.[f]	log k$_1$[g] exp.	log k$_1$[g] calc.[h]
Amphetamine	1.99	9.90	1.78	1.80	-1.12	-0.92	--	--
N-Methyl-	2.21	10.11	1.77	1.77	-1.11	-1.02	-1.925	-1.931
N-Ethyl-	2.73	10.23	1.55	1.61	-1.24	-1.26	-1.784	-1.890
N-n-Propyl-	3.26	9.98	1.40	1.37	-1.41	-1.50	-1.622	-1.585
N-2-Propyl-	3.15	10.14	1.53	1.43	-1.33	-1.45	-1.662	-1.907
N-n-Butyl-	3.79	(9.98)	0.70	1.04	-1.93	-1.75	-1.545	-1.279
N-2-Butyl-	3.67	(10.14)	1.25	1.11	-1.60	-1.69	-1.695	-1.607
N-Benzyl-	3.93	7.50	-0.37	-0.13[i]	-2.77	-1.81[j]	-1.273	-1.198
N,N-Dimethyl-	2.64	9.80	1.53	1.64	-1.23	-1.22	-1.491	-1.683

N,N-Diethyl-	3.70	(9.80)	1.46	1.10	-1.31	-1.71	-1.039	-1.331
N,N-Di-n-propyl-	4.75	(9.80)	0.10	0.19	-1.94	-2.19	-0.772	-0.725
N,N-Di-n-butyl-	5.81	(9.80)	-1.00	-1.08	-3.20	-2.68	0.301	-0.113
N-Methyl-N-ethyl-	3.17	9.80	1.47	1.41	-1.30	-1.46	-1.434[k]	-1.377
							-1.600[l]	-1.636
N-Methyl-N-n-propyl-	3.70	(9.80)	1.27	1.10	-1.44	-1.70	-0.970[k]	-1.071
							-1.478[l]	-1.331
N-Methyl-N-n-butyl-	4.23	(9.80)	0.39	0.69	-2.17	-1.95	-0.851[k]	-0.765
							-1.619[l]	-1.025

[a] Calculated according to Rekker [17].
[b] Values determined by Vree et al. [212]; values in parentheses are estimates.
[c] log percent excreted unchanged.
[d] Calculated from Eq. (40).
[e] log rate constant of renal excretion (hr^{-1}).
[f] Calculated from Eq. (42).
[g] log rate constant of first N-dealkylation step (hr^{-1}).
[h] Calculated from Eq. (44).
[i] Calculated from Eq. (41).
[j] Outlier not included in Eq. (42).
[k] Removal of N-methyl group.
[l] Removal of N-alkyl group.
Source: From Ref. 211.

equation indicates that the rate of dealkylation increases with the partition coefficient and decreases with increasing steric hindrance at C_α. The equation is thus physically meaningful in that it confirms previous discussions, particularly in Secs. IV.B and IV.C.

$$\log EXC = -0.461(\pm 0.018) \log P \tag{42}$$

$$n = 14; \ r^2 = 0.981; \ s = 0.240; \ F = 675$$

$$\log k_1 = 0.537(\pm 0.086) \log P - 3.27(\pm 0.032) \tag{43}$$

$$n = 17; \ r^2 = 0.723; \ s = 0.290; \ F = 39.1$$

$$\log k_1 = 0.577(\pm 0.074) \log P$$

$$+ 0.259(\pm 0.099) \ (\text{number of H atoms on } C_\alpha) - 3.99(\pm 0.38)$$

$$n = 17; \ r^2 = 0.814; \ s = 0.246; \ F = 30.6 \tag{44}$$

VIII. CONCLUSION

In this chapter we have attempted a detailed examination from several viewpoints of the relationships that exist between the chemical structure of molecules and the processes of biotransformation and disposition which they undergo. It is readily apparent that a number of forms of selectivity occur during the course of these processes, and this discrimination depends both on the nature of the biological system concerned and the inherent properties of the drug molecule. Thus, the modulation of the integrity of an enzymic mechanism by the use of inducing agents has clearly been demonstrated to have a marked effect on the way in which biotransformation occurs. On the other hand, small differences in chemical structure may cause marked changes in the ability of drug-metabolizing enzymes to interact with regioisomeric, diastereoisomeric, and enantiomeric substrates. Similarly, it is now clear that the discrimination by enzymes among regiotopic, diastereotopic, and enantiotopic groups in a molecule is of the utmost importance.

The topic we have discussed obviously belongs to the far more extensive and complex subject of structure-activity relationships in biological systems. However, at the present state of our knowledge we can only examine fragments, even though these are complementary, of the overall picture. Our final objective would be to gain a global and comprehensive insight into molecular structure (molecular architecture and molecular properties) in connection with drug metabolism and more generally with any biological response. This overall understanding is, however, still far removed. Indeed, it is necessary first to acquire and analyze much more new data and to devise novel approaches to this topic, as exemplified by QSAR studies, before the thousand facets merge in our understanding to reveal the diamond we yet fail to see.

The achievement of this goal will allow us to show why the biological response elicited by an exogenous molecule may, in some cases, be desirable (drug therapy or pest control), detrimental (toxicological effects such as teratogenesis or mutagenesis), or both depending upon circumstances (as seen in biotransformation processes). Indeed, with further expansion, the predictive value of this kind of work will be considerable, easing the design of novel drug molecules and acting as an invaluable guide to drug development as a whole.

REFERENCES

1. E. L. Eliel, Stereochemistry of Carbon Compounds. McGraw-Hill, New York, 1962, pp. 434-437.
2. W. L. Alworth, Stereochemistry and Its Application in Biochemistry. Wiley, New York, 1972, p. 5.
3. P. S. Portoghese, Ann. Rev. Pharmacol. $\underline{10}$:51 (1970).
4. V. Prelog, Ind. Chem. Belge, p. 1309 (1962).
5. P. Jenner and B. Testa, Drug Metab. Rev. $\underline{2}$:117 (1973).
6. H. R. Bosshard, Experientia $\underline{32}$:949 (1976).
7. K. Dalziel, Phil. Trans. Roy. Soc., Ser. B $\underline{272}$:109 (1975).
8. B. Testa, Drug Metab. Rev. $\underline{5}$:i (1976).
9. B. Testa, Principles of Organic Stereochemistry. Dekker, New York, 1979, pp. vii-ix.
10. B. Testa and P. Jenner, Drug Metabolism: Chemical and Biochemical Aspects. Dekker, New York, 1976, Chaps. 1.4 and 1.5.
11. B. Testa and P. Jenner, J. Pharm. Pharmacol. $\underline{28}$:731 (1976).
12. D. C. Hobbs and H. M. Ilhenny, Ann. Rep. Med. Chem. $\underline{11}$:190 (1976).
13. H. M. Ilhenny, Ann. Rep. Med. Chem. $\underline{12}$:201 (1977).
14. G. Bauer-Staeb and P. Niebes, Experientia $\underline{32}$:367 (1976).
15. A. M. Burkman, R. E. Notari, and W. K. Van Tyle, J. Pharm. Pharmacol. $\underline{26}$:493 (1974).
16. R. W. Fuller, J. C. Baker, and B. B. Molloy, J. Pharm. Sci. $\underline{66}$:271 (1977).
17. R. F. Rekker, The Hydrophobic Fragmental Constant, Its Derivation and Application: A Means of Characterizing Membrane Systems. Elsevier, Amsterdam, 1977.
18. A. K. Cho and G. T. Miwa, Drug Metab. Dispos. $\underline{2}$:477 (1974).
19. S. Safe, D. Jones, and O. Hutzinger, J. Chem. Soc. P.T.I. p. 357 (1976).
20. J. W. Gorrod, Chem. Biol. Interact. $\underline{7}$:289 (1973).
21. P. Hlavica and M. Kehl, Biochem. J. $\underline{164}$:487 (1977).
22. B. Testa and P. Jenner, Drug Metab. Rev. $\underline{7}$:325 (1978).
23. P. A. Cammer and R. M. Hollingworth, Biochem. Pharmacol. $\underline{25}$: 1799 (1976).

24. G. M. Rosen and E. J. Rauckman, Biochem. Pharmacol. 26:675 (1977).
25. G. M. Rosen, E. J. Rauckman, and K. W. Hanck, Toxicol. Lett. 1:71 (1977).
26. J. Kristoffersson, L. Å. Svensson, and K. Tegnér, Acta Pharm. Suec. 11:427 (1974).
27. R. A. Van Dyke and C. G. Wineman, Biochem. Pharmacol. 20:463 (1971).
28. G. Loew, J. Trudell, and H. Motulsky, Mol. Pharmacol. 9:152 (1973).
29. T. Hayakawa, S. Udenfriend, H. Yagi, and D. M. Jerina, Arch. Biochem. Biophys. 170:438 (1975).
30. D. M. Jerina, in Glutathione: Metabolism and Function (I. M. Arias and W. B. Jacobi, eds.). Raven Press, New York, 1976, pp. 267-279.
31. K. B. Jacobson, J. Biol. Chem. 236:343 (1961).
32. A. Poland and E. Glover, Mol. Pharmacol. 13:924 (1977).
33. J. A. Goldstein, P. Hickman, H. Bergman, J. D. McKinney, and M. P. Walker, Chem. Biol. Interact. 17:69 (1977).
34. See Ref. 9, Chap. 4.
35. K. Mislow, Bull. Soc. Chim. Belg. 86:595 (1977).
36. S. B. Matin, S. H. Wan, and J. B. Knight, Biomed. Mass Spectrom. 4:118 (1977).
37. A. Breckenridge and M. L'E. Orme, Life Sci. 11:337 (1972).
38. W. Schmidt and E. Jähnchen, J. Pharm. Pharmacol. 29:266 (1977).
39. E. Jähnchen, T. Meinertz, H. J. Gilfrich, U. Groth, and A. Martini, Clin. Pharmacol. Ther. 20:342 (1976).
40. D. S. Hewick and A. M. M. Shepherd, J. Pharm. Pharmacol. 28:257 (1976).
41. R. A. O'Reilly, Clin. Pharmacol. Ther. 16:348 (1974).
42. D. S. Hewick and J. McEwen, J. Pharm. Pharmacol. 25:458 (1973).
43. A. Yacobi and G. Levy, J. Pharmacokinet. Biopharm. 5:123 (1977).
44. J. A. Gray, H. Lüllmann, F. Mitchelson, and G. H. Reil, Brit. J. Pharmacol. 56:485 (1976).
45. K. Kawashima, A. Levy, and S. Spector, J. Pharmacol. Exp. Ther. 196:517 (1976).
46. A. Levy, S. H. Ngai, A. D. Finck, K. Kawashima, and S. Spector, Eur. J. Pharmacol. 40:93 (1976).
47. C. F. George, T. Fenyvesi, M. E. Conolly, and C. T. Dollery, Eur. J. Clin. Pharmacol. 4:74 (1972).
48. P. J. Murphy, R. C. Nickander, G. M. Bellamy, and W. L. Kurtz, J. Pharmacol. Exp. Ther. 199:415 (1976).
49. L. M. Ball, A. G. Renwick, and R. T. Williams, Xenobiotica 7:101 (1977).
50. Y. Shiobara, Xenobiotica 7:457 (1977).
51. P. Mathieu, J. Greffe, D. Deruaz, R. Guilluy, and L. Gjessing, Biochem. Pharmacol. 25:497 (1976).
52. See Ref. 10, Chap. 1.4.1.

53. W. E. G. Meuldermans, W. F. J. Lauwers, and J. J. P. Heykants, Arch. Int. Pharmacodyn. Thér. 221:140 (1976).
54. J. J. P. Heykants, W. E. G. Meuldermans, L. J. M. Michiels, P. J. Lewi, and P. A. J. Janssen, Arch. Int. Pharmacodyn. Thér. 216:113 (1975).
55. A. Küpfer and J. Bircher, J. Pharmacol. Exp. Ther. 209:190 (1979).
56. C. C. Pfeiffer, Science 124:29 (July 1956).
57. L. G. Dring, R. L. Smith, and R. T. Williams, J. Pharm. Pharmacol. 18:402 (1966).
58. J. Wright, A. K. Cho, and J. Gal, Xenobiotica 7:257 (1977).
59. J. Gal, J. Wright, and A. K. Cho, Res. Commun. Chem. Pathol. Pharmacol. 15:525 (1976).
60. A. Jindra, Jr., O. Heila, and A. Jindra, Experientia 29:395 (1973).
61. H. R. Gutmann and P. Bell, Biochim. Biophys. Acta 498:229 (1977).
62. A. H. Beckett and D. M. Morton, Biochem. Pharmacol. 15:1847 (1966).
63. R. E. Dann, D. R. Feller, and J. F. Snell, Eur. J. Pharmacol. 16: 233 (1971).
64. M. W. Anders, M. J. Cooper, and A. E. Takemori, Drug Metab. Dispos. 1:642 (1973).
65. K. H. Dudley, D. L. Bius, and T. C. Butler, J. Pharmacol. Exp. Ther. 175:27 (1970).
66. K. H. Dudley and D. L. Bius, Drug Metab. Dispos. 4:340 (1976).
67. K. H. Dudley, D. L. Bius, and M. E. Grace, J. Pharmacol. Exp. Ther. 180:167 (1972).
68. K. H. Dudley, T. C. Butler, and D. L. Bius, Drug Metab. Dispos. 2: 103 (1974).
69. R. D. Howland and L. D. Bohm, Biochem. J. 163:125 (1977).
70. I. D. Capel, P. Millburn, and R. T. Williams, Xenobiotica 4:601 (1974).
71. See Ref. 10, Chap. 2.3.1.
72. H. Ehrsson, J. Pharm. Pharmacol. 27:971 (1975).
73. C. D. Arnett, P. S. Callery, and N. Zenker, Biochem. Pharmacol. 26:377 (1977).
74. R. T. Williams, Detoxication Mechanisms, 2nd ed. Chapman & Hall, London, 1959.
75. R. W. Estabrook, G. Martinez-Zedillo, S. Young, J. A. Peterson, and J. McCarthy, J. Ster. Biochem. 6:419 (1975).
76. V. Ullrich, H. H. Ruf, and H. Mimoun, Biochem. Soc. Symp. 34:11 (1972).
77. U. Frommer, V. Ullrich, H. J. Staudinger, and S. Orrenius, Biochim. Biophys. Acta 280:487 (1972).
78. J. N. T. Gilbert, J. W. Powell, and J. Templeton, J. Pharm. Pharmacol. 27:923 (1975).
79. B. K. Tang, T. Inaba, and W. Kalow, Drug Metab. Dispos. 3:479 (1975).

80. W. Kalow, L. Endrenyi, T. Inaba, D. Kadar, and B. Tang, in
    Advances in Pharmacology and Therapeutics (P. Duchene-Murallaz,
    ed.), vol. 6. Pergamon, Oxford, 1979, pp. 31-40.
81. See Ref. 10, Sec. 1.1.1.2.
82. R. E. McMahon and H. R. Sullivan, Life Sci. 5:921 (1966).
83. M. Widman, J. Dahmén, K. Leander, and K. Petersson, Acta Pharm.
    Suec. 12:385 (1975).
84. S. Agurell, M. Binder, K. Fonseka, J. E. Lindgren, K. Leander,
    B. Martin, I. M. Nilsson, M. Nordqvist, A. Ohlsson, and M. Wid-
    man, in Marihuana: Chemistry, Biochemistry, and Cellular Effects
    (G. F. Nahas, ed.). Springer, New York, 1976, pp. 141-157.
85. K. Fonseka and M. Widman, J. Pharm. Pharmacol. 29:12 (1977).
86. W. A. Yisak, M. Widman, J. E. Lindgren, and S. Agurell, J. Pharm.
    Pharmacol. 29:487 (1977).
87. D. J. Harvey, B. R. Martin, and W. D. M. Paton, Biomed. Mass
    Spectrom. 4:364 (1977).
88. L. M. Hjelmeland, L. Aronow, and J. R. Trudell, Mol. Pharmacol.
    13:634 (1977).
89. L. M. Hjelmeland, L. Aronow, and J. R. Trudell, Biochem. Biophys.
    Res. Comm. 76:541 (1977).
90. T. Ishida, Y. Asakawa, M. Okano, and T. Aratani, Tetrahedron
    Lett. p. 2437 (1977).
91. E. Dagne and N. Castagnoli, Jr., J. Med. Chem. 15:356 (1972).
92. B. Lindeke, G. Hallström, E. Andersson, and B. Karlén, Xenobiotica
    7:95 (1977).
93. R. T. Coutts, G. W. Dawson, and A. H. Beckett, J. Pharm. Phar-
    macol. 28:815 (1976).
94. B. Dittmann and G. Renner, N.-S. Arch. Pharmakol. 296:87 (1977).
95. C. Mitona, R. L. Dehn, and M. Tanabe, Biochim. Biophys. Acta
    237:21 (1971).
96. F. M. Belpaire and M. G. Bogaert, Xenobiotica 5:421 (1975).
97. A. W. Burg, Drug Metab. Rev. 4:199 (1975).
98. M. J. Arnaud, Biochem. Med. 16:67 (1976).
99. I. C. Gunsalus, T. C. Pederson, and S. G. Sligar, Ann. Rev. Bio-
    chem. 44:377 (1975).
100. G. A. Hamilton, J. R. Giacin, T. M. Hellman, M. E. Snook, and
     J. W. Weller, Ann. N.Y. Acad. Sci. 212:4 (1973).
101. F. Lichtenberger, W. Nastainczyk, and V. Ullrich, Biochem. Bio-
     phys. Res. Comm. 70:939 (1976).
102. A. D. Rahimtula, P. J. O'Brien, E. G. Hrycay, J. A. Peterson,
     and R. W. Estabrook, Biochem. Biophys. Res. Comm. 60:695 (1974).
103. J. H. Dawson, R. H. Holm, J. R. Trudell, G. Barth, R. E. Linder,
     E. Bunnenberg, C. Djerassi, and S. C. Tang, J. Amer. Chem. Soc.
     98:3707 (1976).
104. R. W. Estabrook and J. Werringloer, in Drug Metabolism Concepts
     (D. M. Jerina, ed.). American Chemical Soc., Washington, D.C.,
     1977, pp. 1-26.

105. B. Testa, J. C. Bünzli, and W. P. Purcell, J. Theor. Biol. 70:339 (1978).
106. H. W. Orf and D. Dolfin, Proc. Nat. Acad. Sci. U.S. 71:2646 (1974).
107. R. E. Keay and G. A. Hamilton, J. Amer. Chem. Soc. 97:6876 (1975).
108. D. B. Northrop, Biochemistry 14:2644 (1975).
109. E. Dagne, L. Gruenke, and N. Castagnoli, Jr., J. Med. Chem. 17: 1330 (1974).
110. M. M. Abdel-Monem, J. Med. Chem. 18:427 (1975).
111. W. A. Garland, S. D. Nelson, and H. A. Sasame, Biochem. Biophys. Res. Comm. 72:539 (1976).
112. I. Björkhem, Pharmacol. Ther. A 1:327 (1977).
113. S. D. Nelson, L. R. Pohl, and W. F. Trager, J. Med. Chem. 18: 1062 (1975).
114. B. Testa, D. Mihailova, and R. Natcheva, Eur. J. Med. Chem. 14: 295 (1979).
115. B. Testa and D. Maihailova, J. Med. Chem. 21:683 (1978).
116. J. A. Pople, Bull. Soc. Chim. Belg. 85:347 (1976).
117. I. G. Csizmadia, Theory and Practice of MO Calculations in Organic Molecules. Elsevier, Amsterdam, 1976, pp. 307-364.
117a. R. S. Mulliken, J. Chem. Phys. 23:1833, 1841 (1955).
118. M. D. Burke and R. T. Mayer, Drug Metab. Dispos. 3:245 (1975).
119. H. G. Selander, D. M. Jerina, and J. W. Daly, Arch. Biochem. Biophys. 168:309 (1975).
120. H. G. Selander, D. M. Jerina, D. E. Piccolo, and G. A. Berchtold, J. Amer. Chem. Soc. 97:4428 (1975).
121. P. E. Thomas, A. Y. H. Lu, D. Ryan, S. B. West, J. Kawalek, and W. Levin, Mol. Pharmacol. 12:746 (1976).
122. L. A. Sternson and R. E. Gammans, Bioorg. Chem. 4:58 (1975).
123. P. J. Meffin and J. Thomas, Xenobiotica 3:625 (1973).
124. C. Stubley, L. Subryan, J. G. P. Stell, R. H. Perrett, P. B. H. Ingle, and D. W. Mathieson, J. Pharm. Pharmacol. 29(Suppl):77P (1977).
125. T. C. Connors, J. A. Hickman, M. Jarman, D. H. Melzack, and W. C. J. Ross, Biochem. Pharmacol. 24:1665 (1975).
126. T. Watabe and T. Sawahata, Biochem. Pharmacol. 25:601 (1976).
127. R. P. Hanzlik, M. Edelman, W. J. Michaely, and G. Scott, J. Amer. Chem. Soc. 98:1952 (1976).
128. See Ref. 10, Chap. 1.2.4.
129. G. Marzullo and A. J. Friedhoff, Life Sci. 17:933 (1975).
130. R. L. Bronaugh, S. E. Hattox, M. M. Hoehn, R. C. Murphy, and C. O. Rutledge, J. Pharmacol. Exp. Ther. 195:441 (1975).
131. H. Hirschmann and K. R. Hanson, J. Org. Chem. 36:3293 (1971).
132. See Ref. 9, Chap. 11.
133. K. R. Hanson, J. Biol. Chem. 250:8309 (1975).
134. K. R. Hanson and I. A. Rose, Acc. Chem. Res. 8:1 (1975).

135. R. E. McMahon, H. R. Sullivan, J. C. Craig, and W. E. Pereira, Jr., Arch. Biochem. Biophys. 132:575 (1969).
136. R. E. Billings, H. R. Sullivan, and R. E. McMahon, Biochemistry 9:1256 (1970).
137. T. C. Butler, K. H. Dudley, D. Johnson, and S. B. Roberts, J. Pharmacol. Exp. Ther. 199:82 (1976).
138. J. H. Poupaert, R. Cavalier, M. H. Claesen, and P. A. Dumont, J. Med. Chem. 18:1268 (1975).
139. R. M. Thompson, J. Beghin, W. K. Fife, and N. Gerber, Drug Metab. Dispos. 4:349 (1976).
140. A. Küpfer, J. Bircher, and R. Preisig, J. Pharmacol. Exp. Ther. 203:493 (1977).
141. H. Sobotka, M. F. Holzman, and J. Kahn, J. Amer. Chem. Soc. 54: 4697 (1932).
142. J. Knabe and C. Urbahn, Justus Liebigs Ann. Chem. 750:21 (1971).
143. D. H. Hutson, Chem. Biol. Interact. 16:315 (1977).
144. W. G. Taylor and R. T. Coutts, Drug Metab. Dispos. 5:564 (1977).
145. H. B. Hucker, A. J. Balletto, S. C. Stauffer, A. G. Zacchei, and B. H. Arison, Drug Metab. Dispos. 2:406 (1974).
146. M. E. Christy, P. S. Anderson, B. H. Arison, D. W. Cochran, and E. L. Engelhardt, J. Org. Chem. 42:378 (1977).
147. N. Chatterjie, J. M. Fujimoto, C. E. Inturrisi, S. Roerig, R. I. H. Wang, D. V. Bowen, F. H. Field, and D. D. Clarke, Drug Metab. Dispos. 2:401 (1974).
148. L. Malspeis, M. S. Bathala, T. M. Ludden, H. B. Bhat, S. G. Frank, T. D. Sokoloski, B. E. Morrison, and R. H. Reuning, Res. Commun. Chem. Pathol. Pharmacol. 12:43 (1975).
149. L. Malspeis, T. M. Ludden, M. S. Bathala, B. E. Morrison, D. R. Feller, and R. H. Reuning, Res. Comm. Chem. Pathol. Pharmacol. 14:393 (1976).
150. S. Roerig, J. M. Fujimoto, R. I. H. Wang, S. H. Pollock, and D. Lange, Drug Metab. Dispos. 4:53 (1976).
151. D. J. Harvey, B. R. Martin, and W. D. M. Paton, J. Pharm. Pharmacol. 29:495 (1977).
152. D. J. Harvey and W. D. M. Paton, J. Pharm. Pharmacol. 29:498 (1977).
153. A. G. Renwick and R. T. Williams, Biochem. J. 129:857 (1972).
154. H. E. May, R. Boose, and D. J. Reed, Biochemistry 14:4723 (1975).
155. R. H. Fish, J. E. Casida, and E. C. Kimmel, Tetrahedron Lett. p. 3515 (1977).
156. K. H. Palmer, M. S. Fowler, M. E. Wall, L. S. Rhodes, W. J. Waddell, and B. Baggett, J. Pharmacol. Exp. Ther. 170:355 (1969).
157. K. H. Palmer, M. S. Fowler, and M. E. Wall, J. Pharmacol. Exp. Ther. 175:38 (1970).
158. J. L. Holtzman and J. A. Thompson, Drug Metab. Dispos. 3:113 (1975).

159. F. I. Carroll and J. T. Blackwell, J. Chem. Soc. Chem. Commun. p. 1616 (1970).
160. P. Jenner, J. W. Gorrod, and A. H. Beckett, Xenobiotica 3:563 (1973).
161. P. Jenner, J. W. Gorrod, and A. H. Beckett, Xenobiotica 3:573 (1973).
162. B. Testa, P. Jenner, A. H. Beckett, and J. W. Gorrod, Xenobiotica 6:553 (1976).
163. J. Booth and E. Boyland, Biochem. Pharmacol. 20:407 (1971).
164. J. F. Whidby and J. I. Seeman, J. Org. Chem. 41:1585 (1976).
165. B. Testa and A. H. Beckett, J. Pharm. Pharmacol. 25:119 (1973).
166. B. Testa, Acta Pharm. Suec. 10:441 (1973).
167. P. Baumann and V. Prelog, Helv. Chim. Acta 41:2362 (1958).
168. H. W. Culp and R. E. McMahon, J. Biol. Chem. 243:848 (1968).
169. C. T. Bedford and D. H. Hutson, Chem. Ind. (London) p. 440 (1976).
170. J. D. McKinney, H. B. Matthews, and N. K. Wilson, Tetrahedron Lett. p. 1895 (1973).
171. L. R. Pohl, R. Bales, and W. F. Trager, Res. Commun. Chem. Pathol. Pharmacol. 15:233 (1976).
172. L. R. Pohl, S. D. Nelson, W. R. Porter, W. F. Trager, M. J. Fasco, F. D. Baker, and J. W. Fenton, II, Biochem. Pharmacol. 25:2153 (1976).
173. L. R. Pohl, W. R. Porter, W. F. Trager, M. J. Fasco, and J. W. Fenton, II, Biochem. Pharmacol. 26:109 (1977).
174. M. J. Fasco, L. J. Piper, and L. S. Kaminsky, Arch. Biochem. Biophys. 182:379 (1977).
175. P. Jenner and B. Testa, Xenobiotica 8:1 (1978).
176. R. F. N. Mills, S. S. Adams, E. E. Cliffe, W. Dickinson, and J. S. Nicholson, Xenobiotica 3:589 (1973).
177. C. J. W. Brooks and M. T. Gilbert, J. Chromatogr. 99:541 (1974).
178. G. J. Vangiessen and D. G. Kaiser, J. Pharm. Sci. 64:798 (1975).
179. S. S. Adams, P. Bresloff, and C. G. Mason, J. Pharm. Pharmacol. 28:256 (1976).
180. D. G. Kaiser, G. J. Vangiessen, R. J. Reischer, and W. J. Wechter, J. Pharm. Sci. 65:269 (1976).
181. K. J. Kripalani, A. Zein El-Abdin, A. V. Dean, and E. C. Schreiber, Xenobiotica 6:159 (1976).
182. A. V. Dean, S. J. Lan, K. J. Kripalani, L. T. DiFazio, and E. C. Schreiber, Xenobiotica 7:549 (1977).
183. S. J. Lan, K. J. Kripalani, A. V. Dean, P. Egli, L. T. DiFazio, and E. C. Schreiber, Drug Metab. Dispos. 4:330 (1976).
184. M. Galli Kienle, M. Anastasia, G. Cighetti, A. Manzocchi, and G. Galli, Eur. J. Biochem. 73:1 (1977).
185. C. Hansch, in Drug Design (E. J. Ariëns, ed.), Vol. 1. Academic Press, New York, 1971, pp. 271-342.

186. W. P. Purcell, G. E. Bass, and J. M. Clayton, Strategy of Drug
     Design: A Molecular Guide to Biological Activity. Wiley, New York,
     1973.
187. C. G. Swain and E. C. Lupton, J. Amer. Chem. Soc. 90:4328 (1968).
188. R. W. Taft, in Steric Effects in Organic Chemistry (M. S. Newman,
     ed.). Wiley, New York, 1956, p. 556.
189. A. Bondi, J. Phys. Chem. 68:441 (1964).
190. L. B. Kier and L. H. Hall, Molecular Connectivity in Chemistry and
     Drug Research. Academic Press, New York, 1976.
191. W. Scholtan, Arzneim.-Forsch. 18:505 (1968).
192. W. J. Jusko and M. Gretch, Drug Metab. Rev. 5:43 (1976).
193. R. F. Rekker, in Biological Activity and Chemical Structure (J. A.
     Keverling Buisman, ed.). Elsevier, Amsterdam, 1977, pp. 107-130.
194. T. Fujita, J. Med. Chem. 15:1049 (1972).
195. R. W. Lucek and C. B. Coutinho, Mol. Pharmacol. 12:612 (1976).
196. D. Sharples, J. Pharm. Pharmacol. 28:100 (1976).
197. C. Hansch, Drug Metab. Rev. 1:1 (1972).
198. C. Hansch, A. R. Steward, and J. Iwasa, J. Med. Chem. 8:868
     (1965).
199. Y. C. Martin and C. Hansch, J. Med. Chem. 14:777 (1971).
200. G. L. Tong and E. J. Lien, J. Pharm. Sci. 65:1651 (1976).
201. B. Testa, to be published.
202. J. B. Houston, D. G. Upshall, and J. W. Bridges, J. Pharmacol.
     Exp. Ther. 189:244 (1974).
203. P. G. C. Douch and H. M. Gahagan, Xenobiotica 7:309 (1977).
204. C. Hansch, A. Leo, S. H. Unger, K. H. Kim, D. Nikaitani, and
     E. J. Lien, J. Med. Chem. 16:1207 (1973).
205. J. Forstova, Z. Sipal, and A. Jindra, Pharmazie 28:397 (1973).
206. G. M. Cohen and G. J. Mannering, Mol. Pharmacol. 9:383 (1973).
207. C. Hansch and W. J. Dunn, J. Pharm. Sci. 61:1 (1972).
208. A. Leo, C. Hansch, and D. Elkins, Chem. Rev. 71:525 (1971).
209. M. Tichy, personal communication (1977); material also presented
     as a poster at the IUPAC-IUPHAR Symposium on Biological Activity
     and Chemical Structure, August 30 - September 2, 1977, Noordwijker-
     hout, The Netherlands.
210. T. D. Yih and J. M. van Rossum, Biochem. Pharmacol. 26:2117
     (1977).
211. M. Donike, R. Iffland, and L. Jaenicke, Arzneim.-Forsch. 24:556
     (1974).
212. T. B. Vree, A. T. J. M. Muskens, and J. M. van Rossum,
     J. Pharm. Pharmacol. 21:774 (1969).

Chapter 3

OXIDATIVE FUNCTIONALIZATION REACTIONS

William F. Trager

Department of Pharmaceutical Sciences
University of Washington
Seattle, Washington

Much of the effort spent in drug metabolism studies has been devoted to functionalization reactions, particularly monooxygenase-mediated oxygenations. The present chapter is aimed at presenting the latest findings on the nature and mode of action of monooxygenases, and the new concepts derived therefrom. These findings and concepts in turn are of considerable value in rationalizing a large body of drug metabolism data.

The chapter opens with an introduction of a historical nature, allowing recent discoveries to be viewed in a proper perspective. The monooxygenases are then considered from a biological and biochemical point of view, with particular emphasis being laid on their organization, multiplicity, and in the reaction cycle of cytochrome P-450.

The main body of the chapter is concerned with oxidative reactions, more specifically carbon atom oxidations. Monooxygenases work by first activating an oxygen atom and then transferring the latter to the substrate. Knowledge on the nature of this activated oxygen is critical for an understanding of oxidative reaction mechanisms, and the concept of oxenoid mechanism is discussed in detail. Several classes of structurally distinct carbon atoms are then taken in turn, and the evidence leading to an understanding of oxidation mechanisms is critically evaluated. The concept of oxene insertion into a C—H bond or a C—C π-bond is a powerful tool for explaining many regio- and stereoselective aspects of drug oxidations, but there are good reasons to believe that a mechanism involving initial hydrogen radical abstraction may be operative in some cases. A conclusion to the chapter discusses the possibility of oxene insertion and hydrogen abstraction being components to varying degrees of a concerted hydroxylation mechanism.

I. INTRODUCTION

The observation by Mueller and Miller in the late 1940s that the in vivo metabolism of the carcinogenic dye 4-dimethylaminoazobenzene could be studied
in vitro using rat liver homogenates signaled the birth of drug metabolism
as an independent discipline that has attracted a broad spectrum of investigators from both the biological and physical sciences [1-3]. Mueller and
Miller demonstrated that their system required nicotinamide-adenine di-
nucleotide phosphate (NADP), molecular oxygen, and both the microsomal
and soluble fractions from the liver preparations. Just a few years later
the group at the National Institutes of Health (NIH) headed by B. B. Brodie
characterized a similar system from rabbit liver also localized in the microsomal fraction and showed that it oxidized a broad spectrum of structurally
diverse drugs [4]. Moreover, they demonstrated that oxidative activity re-
sided in the microsomal fraction and that the requirement for the soluble
fraction could be replaced by either NADPH or an NADPH-generating system.
Thus, the system was highly universal in that it required both oxygen and a
reducing agent, placing it in the mixed-function oxidase classification of
Mason [5]. By this is meant that during the course of oxidation one atom of
an oxygen molecule is transferred to substrate while the second atom undergoes a two-electron reduction and appears as water. This classification was
confirmed by the experiments of Posner et al. [6], who using $^{18}O_2$ demonstrated that in the aromatic hydroxylation of acetanilide by rabbit liver microsomes the source of the oxygen atom appearing in the product, 4-hydroxy-
acetanilide, was molecular oxygen and not water. Further biochemical investigations into the nature of the system led to the discovery of a hemoprotein pigment as a necessary component of the system [7,8]. The hemoprotein
was unusual with respect to other hemoproteins in that a highly specific and
characteristic ultraviolet absorption spectrum could be obtained by the following procedure. A sample of the hemoprotein is first added to a reference
cuvette and a sample cuvette; the material in both cuvettes is then reduced
with either dithionite or NADPH, and the sample cuvette is exposed to carbon

monoxide; finally, the difference spectrum is recorded and a characteristic ultraviolet absorption maximum at 450 nm is obtained. It is this
distinguishing spectral property which has led to the name cytochrome
P-450 for the specific group of enzymes that catalyze microsomal oxidations [9].

Since the publication of these early studies a great deal of effort has
been expended to determine the exact chemical nature of the activated oxygen species transferred to the substrate as well as the specificities, structural properties, and numbers of enzymes involved. In this chapter I will
attempt to summarize what is presently known about the biochemical nature
of the system and then to focus on the mechanism of the oxidation of substrates of various classifications. The main emphasis will center on oxidation at aliphatic and aromatic carbon atoms.

II. BIOCHEMICAL PROPERTIES

Since the primary concern of this chapter is microsomal oxidation, knowledge of the biochemical nature of the enzymes involved is necessary to an
understanding of the mechanisms of the reactions these enzymes catalyze.
Such an understanding is becoming increasingly important because these enzymes are essential to the maintenance of the normal functioning of living
organisms in an environment increasingly contaminated with potentially
lethal substances. That the enzymes themselves sometimes generate toxic
intermediates or end products only underscores their importance and the
importance of understanding the system as a whole and the factors that both
influence and control it.

A. Distribution

The cytoplasm of parenchymal liver cells contains a membranous network
of interconnected channels known as the endoplasmic reticulum. Membranes
of the endoplasmic reticulum are divided into two main types: rough and
smooth. The rough membranes have ribosomes attached to their surface
whereas the smooth membranes do not and are derived from the rough. Ribosomes are the sites of synthesis of both proteins (including various enzymes) and lipids involved in the assembly of membranes. The smooth endoplasmic reticulum, although it remains in physical continuity with the rough
endoplasmic reticulum, is a distinct system with definite characteristics of
its own [10].

Isolation of the endoplasmic reticulum by homogenization and differential centrifugation yields particles called microsomes which appear to reflect
the molecular and functional properties of the intact membrane [11]. In addition to a number of other enzymes microsomes contain two electron transport systems. One is an NADPH-linked system in which cytochrome P-450

reductase is first reduced by NADPH and then transfers reducing equivalents to cytochrome P-450. Cytochrome P-450 in its reduced form next serves as the terminal oxidase for transferring oxygen to the substrate. The system is now known to be heterogeneous and to contain an unknown number of closely related enzymes which catalyze the oxidation of steroids, fatty acids, and xenobiotics. It is this system with which this chapter will be primarily concerned. The second electron transport system comprises NADH as the initial reductant, cytochrome b_5 reductase as the intermediary reductant, and cytochrome b_5 as the terminal oxidase. The function of this latter system is not well understood, but it appears to be involved in fatty acid desaturation and may play an auxiliary role in reactions catalyzed by cytochrome P-450.

Although the liver is the primary organ site for these enzyme systems, cytochrome P-450 is known to also be present and functional in lung, kidney, gut, adrenal cortex, skin, brain, aorta, etc. Indeed it appears that it is probably present in all epithelial tissue in mammals. Moreover cytochrome P-450 is found throughout the animal kingdom and occurs, in insects, plants, and bacteria.

B. Organization

For years the study of the cytochrome P-450 system was impeded by the fact that it is membrane bound and so attempts to solubilize and purify the system invariably led to loss of catalytic activity. A major breakthrough came in 1968 when Lu and Coon [12] reported that an enzyme system from rabbit liver microsomes which catalyzed the ω-hydroxylation of fatty acids in the presence of NADPH and molecular oxygen could be solubilized. The solubilization was achieved using the ionic detergent deoxycholic acid in the presence of glycerol, which protected against the inactivation of cytochrome P-450. Moreover, the solubilized system could be resolved into three components on a diethylaminoethyl(DEAE)-cellulose ion exchange column and retained catalytic activity upon reconstitution [12,13]. The three components of the system were found to be cytochrome P-450, cytochrome P-450 reductase, and a lipid component, namely, phosphatidyl choline. All three components were found to be necessary for maximal activity and appear to have the following functional roles: Cytochrome P-450 reductase transfers reducing equivalents from NADPH to cytochrome P-450. Cytochrome P-450 binds molecular oxygen and substrate; upon reduction it releases one atom of oxygen as water and transfers the second atom to the substrate. The role of lipid is less clear but appears to function as the matrix allowing effective interaction between the reductase and the cytochrome. Since these early reports, much progress has been made in purifying the system [14] and several electrophoretically and catalytically distinct cytochrome P-450's have been isolated [15-26].

The accumulated evidence to date suggests that the distribution of enzymes in the microsomal membrane is heterogeneous, that is, cytochrome P-450 and cytochrome P-450 reductase probably exist in high local concentrations in certain regions of the membrane [27]. Since cytochrome P-450 is present in high concentration in liver microsomes (as much as 15% of total protein in liver microsomes), and since it is present in a concentration 20 to 30 times that of cytochrome P-450 reductase [28], two organizational models have emerged to account for efficient catalysis in view of the seeming discrepancy in stoichiometry. These are (1) the rigid system and (2) the nonrigid system advanced by Franklin and Estabrook [29]. In the rigid system NADPH-cytochrome P-450 reductase is surrounded by a complex of cytochrome P-450 molecules and can only transfer electrons to the cytochrome P-450 molecules constituting that specific complex [30]. In the nonrigid model both NADPH-cytochrome P-450 reductase and cytochrome P-450 are surrounded primarily by phospholipids and have translational mobility. Such a scheme would allow a single reductase molecule to transfer electrons to a large number of cytochrome P-450 molecules [27,31]. Which model, if either, represents the true state of affairs remains to be determined.

C. Multiplicity

It had long been suspected that cytochrome P-450 was really a complex of functionally related enzymes rather than a single species. Indeed this possibility was first suggested in the original publication by Brodie and collaborators [4]. Subsequent evidence for multiplicity was obtained from the differential product profiles that were obtained by prior treatment of experimental animals with either inducing agents such as phenobarbital or 3-methylcholanthrene [32-35], or with inhibitors [36]. The different nature of the monooxygenase system after induction with polycyclic aromatic hydrocarbons such as 3-methylcholanthrene is also indicated by a shift in the Soret band of the difference spectrum from 450 nm to 448 nm, a different pH dependence, and a high affinity for aromatic substrates [37,38].

Definite proof that cytochrome P-450 is in reality a family of related enzymes with different but overlapping specificities resides in the actual physical separation of the enzymes into functionally distinct homogeneous forms. Comai and Gaylor [39] were the first to demonstrate that the hemoprotein could be separated into three distinct forms by column chromatography and that these different forms were induced to different extents by prior treatment of rats with either phenobarbital, ethanol, or 3-methylcholanthrene. Two forms of cytochrome P-450 from both phenobarbital- and 3-methylcholanthrene-treated rats having different spectral and catalytic properties were separated by Ryan et al. [40], whereas Haugen et al. [17] isolated multiple forms of P-450 having different substrate selectivities from phenobarbital-treated rabbits. Since the publication of these initial studies many similar reports have appeared, and the interested reader is referred to a recent review [41].

Reasons as to the possible evolutionary advantage for living organisms to have an environmentally responsive system of multiple enzymes rather than a single enzyme with a near universal substrate specificity have been advanced by Ullrich and Kremers [38]. They argue that, since low substrate selectivity and high affinity are inversely related, an enzyme displaying a broad substrate selectivity must necessarily exhibit low affinity. However, many potentially toxic substances present in the environment such as benzpyrene or DDT are usually present in the body in low concentrations, thus requiring high affinities for their efficient removal. A limited number of more selective enzymes would certainly be more efficient in removing such substances.

The second advantage results from the effects of inducers which increase the steady state concentration of microsomal P-450 by increased synthesis and/or decreased breakdown. It is more economical to produce smaller amounts of more specific enzymes rather than large amounts of a less specific, less efficient enzyme. Such a scheme requires that the inducer induces those enzymes which are effective in catalyzing its own metabolism. This appears to be true for the barbiturates and polycyclic aromatic hydrocarbons.

D. Biochemical Mechanism

Cytochrome P-450 is thought to function through the reaction cycle shown in Fig. 1 [42], in which six steps are apparent.

Step 1: The ferric iron-porphyrin-protein complex (P-450) forms a complex with the substrate R. The interaction is measurable by either ultraviolet (UV) spectrophotometry or electron paramagnetic resonance (EPR). In the case of UV spectrophotometry the binding of the substrate to the enzyme complex perturbs the absorption of the heme moiety in a characteristic manner. Typically one adds the test compound to a suspension of microsomes in the sample cuvette, while the reference cuvette contains a suspension of microsomes without additions. The difference spectrum is then recorded. The types of spectral changes one observes have been classified into three groups: type I, characterized by a maximum at 390 nm and a minimum at about 420 nm; type II, with a minimum at about 390 nm and a maximum between 425 and 435 nm; and reverse type I (modified type II) with a minimum at 390 nm and a maximum at about 420 nm [43]. A type I spectral change is associated with metabolism and probably reflects the enzyme-substrate complex between cytochrome P-450 and the added substrate. Pure type I substrates are usually hydrophobic, lack nonbonded electrons and nucleophilic sites, and are therefore incapable of ligand formation, e.g., cyclohexane. A type II spectral change is generally associated with basic amine

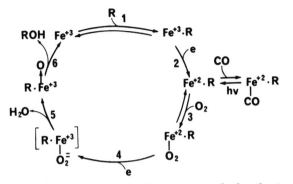

FIGURE 1   The proposed reaction cycle for the transfer of oxene from cytochrome P-450 to substrate.

substrates, e.g., aniline, and is due to ferrihemochrome formation caused by the direct interaction of the heme iron with the nitrogen atom of the substrate [43]. Thus, pure type II substrates generally have nonbonded electrons or nucleophilic sites and are <u>strong ligands</u>, e.g., n-octylamine. Reverse type I spectral changes, which are the mirror image of normal type I, appear to be related to type II, i.e., they arise from similar interactions with the heme iron in degree rather than in kind. Thus, pure reverse type I substrates also have nonbonded electrons and nucleophilic sites but are <u>much weaker ligands</u>, e.g., n-butanol [44].

The ferric iron of cytochrome P-450 has five d electrons in its outer shell, and these electrons can either be paired or unpaired depending upon the state of the enzyme and the nature of the ligands bound to it. In the low spin state (spin 1/2), a single d electron is unpaired and the iron atom has two axial ligands and lies in the plane of the porphyrin ring [45]. This system is characterized by an EPR signal at $g \simeq 2.24$ [46]. In the high spin state, all five d electrons are unpaired and the iron has a single axial ligand and is out of the plane of the porphyrin ring [45]. This system is characterized by an EPR signal at $g \simeq 8.0$ [45]. It has been recognized for some time that the interaction of a type I substrate with cytochrome P-450 is associated with a conversion of hemoprotein from the low spin to the high spin form and that the interaction of a type II compound reflects a conversion of high spin form to low spin form [44]. Recently, a semiquantitative correlation relating spectral changes to changes in spin state has been developed. Indeed, Kumaki et al. [44] have demonstrated that the ratio of the peak heights of the $g \simeq 8.0$ to the $g \simeq 2.24$ EPR signals can be used as a rough measure of the percentage of high spin P-450 iron present in a microsomal sample. Moreover, this study showed that (1) the change from low spin to high spin upon the addition of a type I substrate will cause an increase in the absolute value of the maximum to minimum peak heights in the optical spectrum and that the magnitude of the increase is roughly proportional to the increase of the high spin form; and (2) the change from high spin to low spin upon the addition of either a reverse type I or a type II substrate causes an increase in the absolute value of the maximum to minimum peak heights in the optical spectrum. This increase is presumably roughly proportional to the percentage decrease in high spin form. Thus, if one finds the percentage of high spin form present in intact microsomes prior to the addition of substrate, the degree of change in the optical spectrum produced upon addition of substrate should be predictable.

Step 2: The cytochrome P-450 substrate complex in the ferric oxidation state undergoes a one-electron reduction to the ferrous state [47]. The electron originates from NADPH and is transferred to the complex by cytochrome P-450 reductase.

Step 3: The reduced cytochrome P-450-substrate complex reacts with molecular oxygen to form a tertiary complex [42,48]. Alternatively, the complex can bind carbon monoxide to produce an absorption maximum at about 450 nm. It is this complex formation with carbon monoxide that is responsible for the name cytochrome P-450, as mentioned previously.

Step 4: Oxycytochrome P-450 (Fe^{2+}-O_2-R) undergoes a second one-electron reduction to yield what is effectively a peroxide dianion-substrate-ferric hemoprotein complex. The source of the second electron can be NADPH-cytochrome P-450 reductase or perhaps, at least in vivo, NADH-linked cytochrome b_5 [49,50].

Step 5: Water is released from the complex, resulting in the formation of an oxene intermediate which is the catalytic species that oxidizes the substrate [51]. The oxene intermediate is simply atomic oxygen bound to the ferric hemoprotein and as such is highly electron deficient and therefore a potent oxidizing agent. The nature of this species will form a considerable segment of the discussion to follow.

Step 6: The oxygen atom of the oxene intermediate is transferred to substrate, with subsequent product release from the enzyme complex and return of the iron hemoprotein to the ferric state. Steps 4 and 6 in the overall cycle appear to be rate limiting [48].

III. OXIDATION REACTIONS

Prior to discussing the various classes of oxidations one observes in drug metabolism, a consideration of the nature of the active oxygen species which is transferred to substrate should provide a focus that will help systematize and explain the structural selectivities and regioselectivities that are observed.

A. Nature of Activated Oxygen

In 1964, Hamilton [52] noted the remarkable similarity of many monooxygenase-catalyzed reactions to carbene and nitrene reactions and therefore
suggested that these enzymes catalyze the direct transfer of an oxygen atom
(oxene) to substrate. This transfer he termed the oxenoid mechanism.
    Carbenes ($R_2C:$) and nitrenes ($R\ddot{N}:$) are chemical species which have
only six electrons in the outer valence shell of the carbon or nitrogen atom
and are therefore very reactive by virtue of their electron deficiency. Similarly an oxygen atom (oxene) has only six electrons in its outer valence
shell and hence is isoelectronic with carbene and nitrene. Carbenes will
insert into unactivated carbon hydrogen bonds to give alkanes with overall
retention of configuration, or add to alkenes to give cyclopropanes, or react
with aromatic compounds to give alkylbenzenes and norcaradienes which are
in rapid equilibrium with cycloheptatrienes [53]. The corresponding reactions with oxene would lead (respectively) to alcohols, epoxides, and arene
oxides which are in rapid equilibrium with oxepines, all of which are commonly observed products or known intermediates from microsomal oxidations [54]. Since the reactions of the microsomal monooxygenases resemble
those of singlet (paired nonbonded electrons) rather than those of triplet (two
nonpaired nonbonded electrons) nitrene and carbene, Hamilton concludes
[53] that a free oxygen atom is not involved but rather that an activated enzymic species transfers an oxygen atom to substrate. Indeed, the formation
of a free singlet oxygen atom from a triplet oxygen molecule would be ex-
cessively endothermic and therefore energetically not feasible. Three activated enzymic species that could serve as oxene transfer reagents appear
to be possible: (1) an enzyme-Fe^+-O_2 complex; (2) an enzyme-Fe^{3+}-per-
oxide compound; and (3) an enzyme-Fe^{3+}-O complex. It is important to
recognize that in the structure of these complexes only a single resonance
structure is given and that, for example, the Fe^{3+}-O complex could as
equally well be written as Fe^{4+}-O^- or Fe^{5+}-O^{2-}, as will sometimes be seen
in the literature. Of the three possible structures, Hamilton originally favored the enzyme-Fe^{3+}-peroxide compound as the most probable [53]. However, evidence is now accumulating which suggests that the enzyme-Fe^{3+}-O
complex is probably the active form of oxygen in cytochrome P-450-mediated
reactions.
    In 1974 Rahimtula and O'Brien [55] made the critical observation that
cumene hydroperoxide is capable of supporting the aromatic hydroxylation
of a variety of compounds in the presence of hepatic microsomes. NADPH
and molecular oxygen were not required for the reaction to proceed and
cytochrome P-450 could not be replaced as catalyst by other hemoproteins.
The reactions displayed one-to-one stoichiometry in that one mole of hydroperoxide was consumed for every mole of substrate being hydroxylated.
Moreover, the addition of hydroperoxide to liver microsomes caused the
appearance of both a transient spectral change and the unique electron

paramagnetic resonance signals associated with cytochrome P-450 [56].
The authors therefore concluded that the oxenoid species of cytochrome P-450
was involved in the hydroxylation and that it was present in a form equivalent
to ferryl iron, i.e., $Fe^{4+}-O^-$. Subsequently other investigators have reported that in addition to cumene hydroperoxide various other organic hydro-
peroxides as well as certain inorganic oxidizing agents, e.g., $NaIO_4$ and
H_2O_2, will support hydroxylation reactions catalyzed by P-450 in the absence
of NADPH and O_2 [56-59]. To provide evidence that the active oxygen species involved a ferric cytochrome containing a <u>single oxygen atom</u> and not a
Fe^{3+}-peroxide compound, Lichtenberger et al. [60] studied the O-dealkylation of 7-ethoxycoumarin catalyzed by cytochrome P-450 in the presence of
iodosobenzene (I). They found that iodosobenzene would not only support the

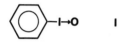

I

O-dealkylation reaction but did so at a rate seven times greater than that
catalyzed by NADPH and O_2 with microsomes from 3-methylcholanthrene-
treated animals. Thus the weight of evidence to date suggests that oxidations
catalyzed by P_{450} can best be viewed as oxene transfer reactions in which
a single oxygen atom bonded to the catalyst is transferred to the substrate.

B. Aliphatic Hydroxylation

If we accept the idea that oxene is the active species of oxygen which is
transferred to the substrate, then the transfer can occur in at least two distinct ways: (1) the oxygen in a single step can simply be inserted into the
bond (e.g., carbon-hydrogen) being functionalized or (2) it can react in a
stepwise fashion. Fortunately the stereochemical consequences of the two
mechanisms are different and therefore are potentially distinguishable. If
the transfer occurs in a single step, i.e., oxygen is inserted directly into
the carbon-hydrogen bond in aliphatic oxidations, one would expect 100% retention of configuration in analogy to singlet carbene reactions. If, on the
other hand, a stepwise process were involved such that an intermediate
radical or a carbonium ion were developed, one would expect at least partial
loss of the stereochemical integrity at the site of metabolic transformation.
The latter possibility now appears to be the case for at least one aliphatic
substrate. Studies using selectively deuterated substrates have presented
compelling evidence that the oxidation of norbornane (II) to norborneol (III)
by a reconstituted rabbit liver cytochrome P-450 system (phenobarbital-
induced, $P-450_{LM2}$) is subject to a very large isotope effect $(k_H/k_D = 11.5 \pm 1)$

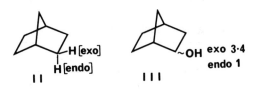

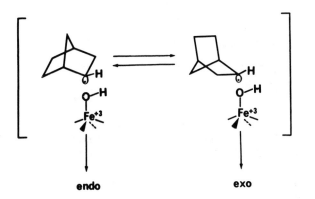

and a significant amount of epimerization [61]. These results are consistent with hydrogen abstraction as the rate-determining step, leading to an intermediate carbon radical which undergoes partial epimerization in the enzyme-substrate cage (Scheme 1). Whether or not such a stepwise mechanism

SCHEME 1

represents the norm in hydroxylations or is an isolated case remains to be determined.

The results obtained in microsomal hydroxylations can be gainfully rationalized by analogy to reactions of carbene or oxenoid (e.g., peroxytri-fluoroacetic acid) reagents. For example, both reagents are selective for tertiary carbon-hydrogen bonds (i.e., tertiary > secondary > primary), and thus in microsomal reactions as a first approximation one expects to find preferential hydroxylation at tertiary and secondary rather than at primary sites in substrates where multiple sites are available. In accord with these expectations are the quantitative hydroxylation patterns obtained using rat liver microsomes for the simple hydrocarbons 2-methylbutane, n-pentane, and n-heptane (Table 1) [62-64]. In addition to the expected regioselectivity, a preference for hydroxylation at the methylene carbon atom adjacent to the terminal carbon is readily apparent. This is a well-recognized phenomenon in drug metabolism and is termed $(\omega-1)$-hydroxylation. Thus, as a general rule, aliphatic substrates or substrates containing side chains

TABLE 1
Microsomal Oxidation of Aliphatic Hydrocarbon Substrates

	Products: alcohols (%)			
Substrate	1	2	3	4
2-Methylbutane: $\overset{1}{C}H_3\overset{3}{C}H(\overset{1}{C}H_3)\overset{2}{C}H_2\overset{1}{C}H_3$	6	20	74	--
n-Pentane: $\overset{3}{C}H_3\overset{2}{C}H_2\overset{1}{C}H_2CH_2CH_3$	0.5	84	16	--
n-Heptane: $\overset{4}{C}H_3\overset{3}{C}H_2\overset{2}{C}H_2\overset{1}{C}H_2CH_2CH_2CH_3$	9.5	73.8	11.1	5.6

Source: Data from Refs. 62-64.

(e.g., barbiturates) would be expected to be regioselective for (ω-1)-hydroxy-
lation. It must be realized, however, that this is merely a general rule and
the situation is greatly complicated by the fact that cytochrome P-450 is a
complex mixture of an undetermined number of enzymes that differ in their
substrate and product selectivities to varying degrees. For example, ω-
hydroxylation is either the major or a significant metabolic pathway for me-
dium chain length (10-18) hydrocarbons and fatty acids [65].

Oxidation of alicyclic compounds should in principle be no different to
the oxidation of open-chain aliphatic substrates. In general this appears to
be the case, as shown by the in vitro metabolism of methylcyclohexane
(Table 2) [63]. Of note is the substantial hydroxylation at C-1, the site of
the tertiary carbon-hydrogen bond, and the minor amount of ω-hydroxylation.
The reason for the apparent selectivity for methylene hydroxylation at C-3
and C-4 over C-2 is not known but does not appear to be an isolated observation in monosubstituted cyclohexanes [65]. Perhaps the product regioselectivity merely reflects the greater steric hindrance at C-2 relative to either
C-3 or C-4 in such a system.

C. Benzylic Hydroxylation

The greater reactivity of a benzylic carbon atom relative to an aliphatic carbon atom is a well-recognized fact in organic chemistry. Resonance stabilization of either radical or carbonium ion intermediates presumably accounts
for this increased reactivity; therefore reactions involving intermediates of
such type in their transition states would be expected to proceed with relative ease. Numerous examples of benzylic hydroxylation catalyzed by

TABLE 2
Microsomal Oxidation of Methylcyclohexane

Substrate		Products: alcohols (%)				
		1	2	3	4	CH$_3$
Methylcyclohexane:	(structure)	25	8	43	23	1

Source: From Ref. 63.

microsomal P-450 can be found in the literature and as such appear to be a common and favored process. This would suggest on first approximation that these reactions are proceeding via a radical or carbonium ion mechanism and therefore that they should display a significant primary isotope effect, assuming cleavage of the carbon hydrogen/deuterium bond to be rate-determining. Further they would be expected to be modulated by resonance effects and should be subject to racemization at the benzylic carbon if it is initially asymmetric.

Conversely benzylic hydroxylation could proceed by a direct insertion mechanism. If this occurs one would expect the reaction to occur by front-side attack with a high degree of retention of configuration. Such a mechanism would also be expected to display a primary isotope effect of relatively low magnitude for two reasons: first, such a mechanism does not really involve bond breaking in the extreme sense; second, such a mechanism requires a "triangular" transition state, a condition which will necessarily lead to a small isotope effect [66].

Probably the study most often cited with regard to benzylic hydroxylation is that of McMahon and collaborators [67], who investigated the metabolism of ethylbenzene using 15,000g hepatic supernatant (i.e., containing both microsomal and soluble fractions) from normal and phenobarbital-treated rats. By employing (S)-(+)-α-d-ethylbenzene (IV) and α,α-d$_2$-ethylbenzene as substrates, it was demonstrated that the reactions with control supernatant proceeded by frontside attack to generate (R)-(+)-2-d-methyl phenyl carbinol (V) with a high degree (86%) of retention of configuration and

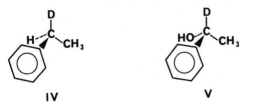

IV   V

à small isotope effect ($k_H/k_D = 1.8$). These results are exactly what would
be expected from a direct insertion or singlet carbene-type reaction. These
workers also reported that when phenobarbital-induced supernatant was uti-
lized as the source of enzymes the degree of retention was much less (ca.
65%), suggesting that perhaps either a qualitatively or quantitatively altered
enzyme mix could account for the decreased product stereoselectivity.

In a subsequent study Billings and coworkers [68] investigated the benzylic hydroxylation of indan (VI) to 1-indanol (VII) and further oxidation to
indanone (VIII). The results showed that the indanol produced was either

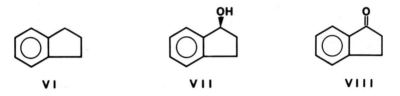

V I   **V I I**   **V I I I**

racemic (microsomes) or enriched in the (S)-(+)-isomer (15,000g supernatant) and that its optical purity was inversely related to the amount of indanone formed concomitantly. Since the oxidation of indanol to indanone was
shown to be substrate stereoselective for the (S)-(+)-isomer, the initial oxidation of indan to indanol was deduced to be even more product stereoselective for the (S)-(+)-isomer than calculated.

In order to clarify the reduced product stereoselectivity found after
phenobarbital induction, Maylin and associates [69] reinvestigated the oxidation of ethylbenzene. In their study they employed both a 9000g supernatant fraction and the 105,000g pellet. The former preparation was found
to oxidize (S)-(-)-methyl phenyl carbinol to acetophenone at a slightly faster
rate than the (R)-enantiomer and in addition contained a reductase which
would reduce with product stereoselectivity the acetophenone so generated
back to the (S)-(-)-carbinol. Upon treatment with phenobarbital the rate of
oxidation of ethylbenzene to the carbinol as well as to acetophenone was
markedly enhanced while the substrate stereoselectivity of the oxidation to
acetophenone was slightly decreased. The product stereoselectivity of the
reduction, however, was unaffected by phenobarbital treatment. Thus the
enhanced rate of oxidation of both ethylbenzene and 1-phenylethanol provides
an increased amount of acetophenone for reduction by the soluble reductase
to (S)-(-)-1-phenylethanol, thereby reducing the overall enantiomeric ratio.
These observations therefore would appear to provide a nice explanation for
why McMahon et al. [67] observed less product stereoselectivity after phenobarbital treatment. However, this conclusion is considerably clouded if one
considers the data presented in Figure 5 of the paper by Maylin et al. [69].
In that figure the enantiomeric composition of the 1-phenylethanols formed
from ethylbenzene is reported as a function of time and source of enzyme.
The results indicate that the enantiomeric composition in experiments with

the 9000g supernatant was not only richer in the (R)-enantiomer <u>after, rather</u> <u>than before</u> phenobarbital pretreatment (as found by McMahon et al.), <u>but</u> <u>increased</u> as a function of time. Perhaps even more significant is the fact that the microsomal fraction from both control and phenobarbital-pretreated animals was product stereoselective for the formation of <u>(S)-(-)-1-phenyl-</u> <u>ethanol</u>. Thus, it would appear that the issue is far from resolved, and fur- ther work is required before any definitive conclusions can be reached re- garding the mechanism of hydroxylation.

Benzylic hydroxylation, although electrophilic in nature, probably in- volves a radical intermediate [61] just as occurs in aliphatic hydroxylation. In an elegant study by Hjelmeland and colleagues, hydroxylation of a series of substituted 1,3-diphenylpropanes [(IX, X, and XI); x = H, F, CH$_3$, or CF$_3$]

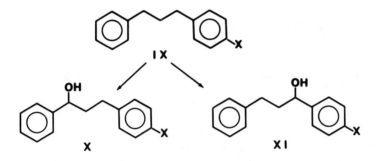

was investigated with respect to the electronic nature of the reaction [70]. The substrates were specifically designed to provide a system in which oxi- dation can occur at either of two electronically different but sterically equi- valent sites. Since only one molecule is involved, the potential problem of differences in binding due to different substituents is eliminated. Moreover, because of the intramolecular competition for hydroxylation sites in such a system, analysis of product distribution can replace the measurement of enzymic velocities as the primary observation, thereby circumventing the effects of other potential, partially rate-determining steps (e.g., binding or P-450 reduction) in the overall sequence. This in hard terms means that effects on the <u>single step</u> of substrate oxidation can be determined [71]. The results (Table 3) clearly demonstrate that the most electron-rich benzylic site is the favored site for hydroxylation. The authors of this study conclude that the results are clearly consistent with an electrophilic mechanism but that the observed regioselectivity is lower than expected for reactions having fully developed carbonium ion character in the transition state.

Since their system is ideally suited to measure effects on the isolated hydroxylation step itself Hjelmeland et al. [72] extended their studies to in- clude 1,3-diphenylpropane-1,1-d$_2$ as substrate. Such a system should pro- vide a measure of the "true" primary isotope effect, that is, a measure of

TABLE 3
Competitive Microsomal Hydroxylation of Substituted
Diphenylpropanes (IX)

Substituent	σ[a]	Product formed (%)	
		X	XI
H	0	50	50
F	0.06	70	30
CH_3	-0.17	50	50
CF_3	0.54	95	5

[a] Hammett sigma value of substituent.
Source: From Ref. 70.

the effect of deuterium substitution on the rate of the specific step involving covalent modification of the substrate. In contrast to the low values (k_H/k_D of about 2.0) that are generally found for hydroxylation reactions catalyzed by P-450, the authors found a large k_H/k_D value of 11 for their system. Based on these results they suggest that a radical abstraction-recombination mechanism be considered as a possible mechanism for benzylic hydroxylation. Certainly the magnitude of the isotope effect is consistent with this hypothesis, and it would be both interesting and informative to investigate how this magnitude is affected by electron-donating and electron-withdrawing para-substituents. In addition, the microsomal hydroxylation of 1,3-diphenylpropane may be highly product stereoselective due to the prochirality of the benzylic centers. To my knowledge, however, the stereochemistry of the reaction has not been determined, although such a study would add significantly to our understanding of the mechanism.

In this regard it is noteworthy that radical abstraction for benzylic moieties was postulated several years ago to explain the unusual toxicity of benzyl alcohol and the seemingly special characteristics of benzylic and allylic moieties in biochemical processes [73].

D. Oxidation Adjacent to Heteroatoms

A very common and general reaction found in drug metabolism is the cytochrome P-450-catalyzed removal of alkyl groups bonded to heteroatoms, in particular oxygen and nitrogen. Since this topic is discussed at length elsewhere in this work (see Chap. 2) it will not be covered in any significant depth here except to draw correlations to the subject matter already discussed.

Although controversial for a considerable period of time it is now generally accepted that the first step in the reaction leading to dealkylation is
the formation of a carbinolamine in the case of nitrogen (presumably a hemi-
acetal in the case of oxygen) which subsequently rearranges to a secondary
amine (alcohol) and aldehyde (Scheme 2). Whether the initial formation of
the carbinolamine proceeds by direct insertion or hydrogen abstraction followed by the addition of a hydroxyl radical is not known and may in fact contain elements of both possibilities.

$$R_2NCH_2CH_3 \longrightarrow R_2NCHOHCH_3 \longrightarrow R_2NH + CH_3CHO$$

SCHEME 2

In a study of the microsomal N-dealkylation of the antiarrhythmic
agent lidocaine (XII) in our laboratory we found both a small primary isotope effect ($k_H/k_D = 1.49$) and a relatively large secondary isotope effect

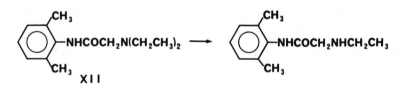

$(k_H/k_D = 1.52)$ [74]. On the assumption that the observed isotope effect
reflected the bond-breaking step we interpreted the results to mean an
asymmetric and/or nonlinear transition state was involved in the removal
of the hydrogen and that the carbon atom being affected had considerable
sp^2-like character in the transition state.

Thus a transition state (XIII) incorporating these properties was postulated wherein the complex formed a two-electron, three-center bond with

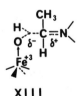

oxene insertion. The results of Abdel-Monem [75] are consistent with this
hypothesis, since the microsomal N-demethylation of 1-(N-methyl-N-tri-
deuteriomethylamino)-3-phenylpropane (XIV) proceeds with an isotope effect
giving $k_H/k_D = 1.3$ as determined by product ratio analysis. This system

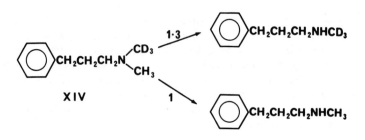

XIV

should be a measure of the "true isotope" effect involved in the bond-breaking step as discussed earlier [71, 72]. Thus, the observation of a small isotope effect supports the idea that the nonbonded electrons on nitrogen are
involved in some fashion in stabilization of the transition state but does not
exclude the possibility of a simple direct insertion. The significant secondary isotope effect observed in the case of lidocaine would argue against
a simple direct insertion if it were firmly established that the effect was
arising solely from the bond-breaking step by intramolecular competition
studies.

Several years ago the hypothesis was advanced that the microsomal
demethylation of tertiary amines involves the initial radical abstraction of
a hydrogen atom [76] (Scheme 3). Later it was suggested [73] that the unusual stabilizing effect of elements such as nitrogen or oxygen could best be
accounted for in terms of Linnett's double quartet theory and symbolism [77,
78] (Scheme 4). Thus, a rate-determining step involving initial abstraction

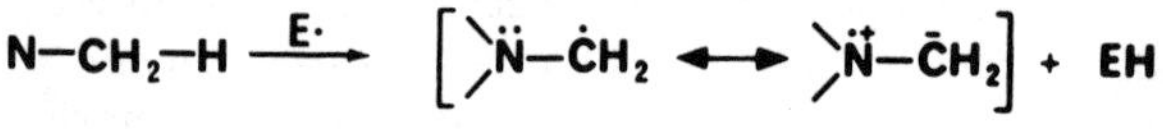

$$N-CH_2-H \xrightarrow{\text{E·}} \left[\overset{..}{N}-\dot{C}H_2 \longleftrightarrow \overset{..}{N}-\bar{C}H_2 \right] + EH$$

SCHEME 3

$$\overset{\cdot}{N} \div \dot{C}H_2$$
$$\tfrac{1}{2}^{+} \quad \tfrac{1}{2}^{-}$$

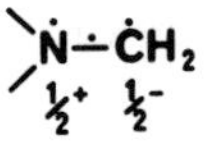

SCHEME 4

of a hydrogen atom by oxene to generate a hydroxyl radical-Fe^{3+} complex
and a Linnett stabilized methylene radical followed by a rapid transfer of
the hydroxyl radical to the methylene radical and generation of ferric cytochrome P-450 would be consistent with all the results discussed thus far
(Scheme 5).

Nevertheless it should be realized that a carbonium ion mechanism is
equally consistent with the data. Thus the reaction could proceed by abstraction of a hydride ion by oxene to generate an iminium ion and a hydroxyl

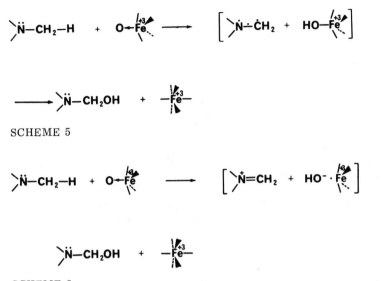

SCHEME 5

SCHEME 6

anion-Fe^{3+} complex (Scheme 6). This sequence could be followed by rapid transfer of the hydroxyl anion back to the iminium ion, forming a carbinolamine and ferric cytochrome P-450. The evidence on norbornane [61] and on 1,3-diphenylpropane [70] strongly suggests a radical mechanism. However, there is evidence from the author's laboratory [79,80] and from other studies [81-84] that iminium ions are in fact intermediates in N-dealkylation reactions. Since the time sequence for their formation is not known, that is, whether they are formed by initial abstraction of hydride as shown in Scheme 6 or whether they are formed from the carbinolamine intermediate by the elimination of water, the question as to the exact mechanism of their formation remains an open one.

Isotope effects for O-dealkylation, like N-dealkylation, are generally found in the range of 1-2. For example, the O-demethylation of ortho-nitroanisole-d3(methyl), para-nitroanisole-d3(methyl), or para-[methyl-d2]acetanilide and the O-dealkylation of para-[1,1-d2]ethoxy-acetanilide proceed with k_H/k_D values of ca. 2 [85], 1.85 [86], 1.90 [86], and 1.61 [87], respectively. In one case of which the author is aware, where an isotope effect was determined for O-demethylation by an intramolecular competition experiment, an effect giving $k_H/k_D = 10$ was observed. Indeed, the methyl group in para-trideuteromethoxyanisole (XV) was oxidatively cleaved at a rate 10 times greater than the trideuteromethyl group, as measured by mass spectrometry and product analysis [86].

In contrast, measuring the rate of O-demethylation of para-dimethoxy-benzene versus para-di(trideuteromethoxy)benzene yielded a k_H/k_D value of

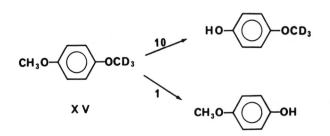

only 2. Clearly the intramolecular competition experiment is superior in giving a true measure of the isotope effect in the bond-breaking step and, together with the second experiment, illustrates that other factors are important in determining the overall rate of reaction. Moreover, the illustration of such a large isotope effect argues against direct insertion and is strong evidence for a radical (hydride) abstraction-recombination mechanism.

E. Aromatic Hydroxylation

The oxidation of aromatic hydrocarbons to phenols at least theoretically can occur by a number of different mechanistic steps [88]. These are (i) abstraction, (ii) insertion, (iii) direct addition, and (iv) addition-rearrangement (Scheme 7). Experimentally determinable criteria for each of the four possible mechanisms may be outlined as follows:

    i. Abstraction
        a. If the substrate is labeled with an isotope in the position that becomes hydroxylated, it will be lost in the formation of product.
        b. The existence of a nonradical or nonionic intermediate between substrate and product is impossible (the isolation of an ionic salt might be possible depending upon the chemical nature of the substrate).
        c. A primary isotope effect will be observed if the substrate is suitably labeled.
   ii. Insertion into carbon-hydrogen bond
        a. Same as item i.
        b. No intermediates are possible.
        c. A primary isotope effect of low magnitude will be observed.
  iii. Direct addition to a carbon-carbon aromatic bond
        a. Label may be retained in the product.
        b. An arene oxide intermediate may exist and be sufficiently stable to be isolated depending upon the chemical nature of the substrate, or its existence might be inferred by the formation of secondary products through reaction with suitable (nucleophilic) trapping agents.
        c. A primary isotope effect will not be observed.

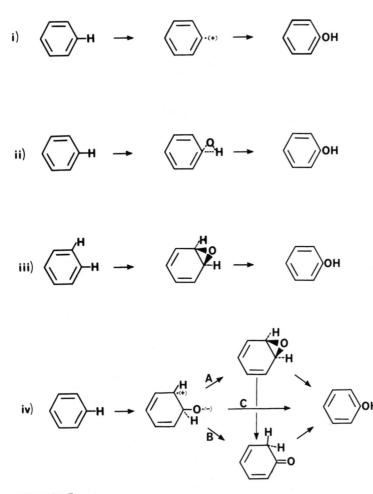

SCHEME 7

    iv. <u>Addition–rearrangement</u>
        a. Label may be retained in the product, path A or B, but not C.
        b. Either the existence (A and B) or nonexistence (C) of isolable
            intermediates may be determined.
        c. The presence (C) or absence of a primary isotope effect (A and
            B) may be demonstrated.

Since arene oxides have been isolated [89–91] and in general isotopic labels are retained with no observable isotope effects, the formation of phenols from aromatic hydrocarbons is now widely accepted as occurring by a direct

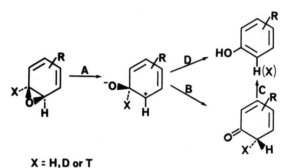

X = H, D or T

SCHEME 8

addition to a carbon-carbon aromatic bond. Moreover, the direct addition
pathway is precisely the pathway expected if the enzymic oxidizing agent
functions by an oxenoid mechanism (Scheme 8). Under physiological conditions the rate-limiting step for the subsequent rearrangement of the arene
oxide to the phenolic end product is the heterolytic cleavage of the carbon-
oxygen bond to form a carbonium ion (Scheme 8, path A) [88,92]. The carbonium ion either isomerizes to the keto tautomer of the phenol (path B) with
concomitant migration of X as an anion to the electron-deficient center or X
leaves as a cation allowing direct formation of the phenol (path D). As indicated in Scheme 8, path A → B leads to the initial migration of X while
enolization path B → C leads to retention of the migrating substituent (NIH
shift) owing to the selective loss of a proton over other isotopic hydrogen
(deuterium, tritium) species. Conversely, path A → D leads to loss of
X. The degree of retention of X (A → B → C) is dependent upon the nature
of substituents present in the substrate. For monosubstituted benzene substrates, retention is a function of the ability of the substituent to neutralize
the intermediary carbonium ion. In general, those substituents which can
best neutralize the carbonium ion lead to the lower level of retention. This
is particularly true for ionizable substituents in which the anion of the conjugate base is directly conjugated to the site of positive charge. For example, substituents such as OH, NH_2, $NHCOCH_3$, or $NHSO_2Ph$ lead to retention of deuterium in the range of 0-30%, whereas nonionizable substituents
such as -OMe, OPh, Me, CN, NO_2, Cl, Br, F, $CONH_2$ lead to retention of
deuterium in the range of 40-65% (Scheme 9) [93]. Substituents also direct
the opening of the arene oxides to the carbonium ion and therefore control
the position of hydroxylation. As would be anticipated, the oxide opens to
generate the most stable carbonium ion. For example, microsomal hydroxylation of toluene leads to 2- and 4-hydroxytoluene but not 3-hydroxytoluene
[93,94]. In agreement with these results, chemical isomerization of the
three possible toluene oxides leads exclusively to either 4-hydroxytoluene
or 2-hydroxytoluene (Scheme 10).

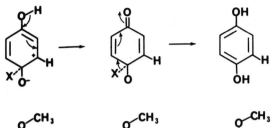

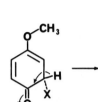

X = H, D or T

SCHEME 9

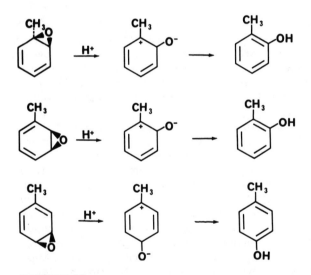

SCHEME 10

Studies of this type or of more highly substituted systems have led to the formulation of a general rule which states that the transition state which contains the greatest number of canonical structures having tertiary carbonium ion character will be favored. For example, the 4,5-oxide of meta-xylene can open in two possible ways, path A or path B. Clearly path B would be the expected pathway, with the resultant formation of 2,4-dimethyl-phenol (Scheme 11). This is indeed what is observed [94].

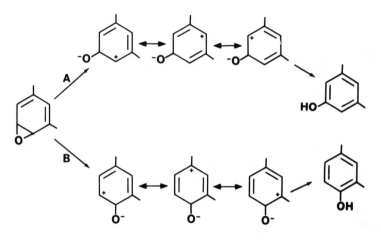

SCHEME 11

As indicated earlier, enough evidence has now been obtained to permit us to conclude that the formation of arene oxide intermediates in microsomal hydroxylation reactions is a general phenomenon. Although the best evidence for such a reaction pathway is the actual isolation of the epoxide itself, the chemical reactivity of such species usually precludes the direct demonstration of their existence via physical isolation. Exceptions include polycyclic aromatic substrates, for example, naphthalene, the epoxide of which has been isolated after incubation with microsomal preparations [95]. Fortunately, there are a number of secondary and experimentally verifiable criteria as outlined earlier by which the production of arene oxides can be inferred: (1) occurrence of the NIH shift, that is, retention of isotopic label in the product, or the migration and retention of substituents such as halogen atoms or alkyl groups (hydroxylating agents which are sources of hydroxyl radical or triplet oxygen do not produce the NIH shift [52,96]); (2) characterization of directly derived metabolites such as dihydrodiols and glutathione conjugates; (3) occurrence in phenolic metabolites of high ortho plus para versus meta ratios, since the opening of the epoxide ring is rate-limiting and will preferentially open to give the most stable carbocation; and (4) observation of negligible or nonexistent isotope effects, since cleavage of a carbon-hydrogen (deuterium, tritium) bond is not involved in the rate–determining step.

Although the intermediacy of arene oxides in microsomal aromatic hydroxylation is a well–established and accepted phenomenon for the vast majority of such reactions, there is evidence for the existence of a subgroup of cytochrome P-450's which are product regioselective for meta-hydroxylation and which, due to this selectivity, are believed to operate by a different mechanism. The existence of such a subgroup of enzymes, if definitively confirmed, will have profound implications in drug metabolism and toxicology since a way would be open to circumvent the cytotoxic and carcinogenic problems associated with arene oxide intermediates.

In 1975, Tomaszewski et al. [88] reported that the in vitro meta-hydroxylation of nitrobenzene and methyl phenyl sulfone was associated with a significant isotope effect (k_H/k_D of 1.40 and 1.75, respectively), whereas the ortho and/or para hydroxylation of the same substrates did not give rise to observable effects. These results indicate that the various hydroxylation pathways are under different enzymic control and that meta-hydroxylation cannot proceed via an arene oxide but is most consistent with a direct insertion of oxene across the carbon-hydrogen bond or with a radical addition-rearrangement pathway.

In an extensive study on the metabolism of chlorobenzene utilizing perfused rat livers, postmitochondrial supernatant, microsomes, and reconstituted soluble hemoprotein systems as the source of P-450 enzymes, all three possible phenolic metabolites (ortho-, meta-, and para-chlorophenol) were found to be produced to a significant extent [97]. However, the relative amount of the meta-isomer was found to decrease with increasing resolution of the hemoprotein-monooxygenase system. Utilization of various inhibitors and inducing agents led to the conclusion that each of the three isomeric products was formed by an independent enzyme. Since 2,3-chlorobenzene oxide was found to isomerize exclusively to ortho-chlorophenol, the occurrence of meta-chlorophenol was interpreted as being the result of a direct oxidative pathway not involving an arene oxide intermediate.

Earlier work on this substrate had demonstrated that not only was meta-chlorophenol a major metabolite [98] but that its formation proceeded without a significant isotope effect (k_H/k_D of 1.17 ± 0.11) [88] and with a relatively low degree of deuterium retention (ca. 24%) [99]. Although the latter experiments were done in vivo and therefore must be interpreted with caution, a radical addition-rearrangement pathway would appear to be the only mechanism consistent with all the results.

In a somewhat analogous study the meta-hydroxylation of biphenyl was found to be species-dependent, to result from an enzymic process distinct from that effecting ortho- and para-hydroxylation, and to proceed with a significant isotope effect, i.e., k_H/k_D of 1.27-1.45 (±0.009-0.069) [100].

As a final example, 7-hydroxylation of the anticoagulant warfarin (XVI) is the major metabolic reaction in humans [101] and the rat, both in vivo [102] and in vitro [103]. Hydroxylation at this site corresponds to meta-hydroxylation and has been demonstrated to occur by an enzymic process distinct from those leading to the 6- and 8-hydroxy metabolites (para- and ortho-hydroxylation, respectively) [103]. The magnitude of the isotope effect associated with 7-hydroxylation, although critical to an understanding of the reaction mechanism, has not as yet been determined.

administration of compounds conjugated with sulfate. What are the implications of this for the synthesis of macromolecules in connective tissues where sulfation is important? In view of the utilization for conjugation of a number of essential compounds, including high-energy nucleotides, alterations of intermediary metabolism as suggested above might well be expected to occur.

Individual variations in susceptibility to disease could also result from variations in conjugative capacity. Several examples of xenobiotic toxicity arising in this way have been quoted, but it is frequently suggested that many diseases have their origin in unrecognized exposure to foreign compounds in the environment, or even faulty metabolism of endogenous toxic compounds. It is interesting to note here that as well as being at risk from drug-induced systemic lupus erythematosus (see Sec. III.A), slow acetylators are also predisposed toward spontaneous lupus erythematosus [117]. This may be due to unrecognized toxic aromatic amines in the environment or to endogenous toxins which undergo acetylation. In either event the finding has important implications for this and other conjugation reactions.

The division of the reactions involved in xenobiotic metabolism into two phases is a useful one but very arbitrary. The two phases should not be considered separately, and without a proper appreciation of the significance of conjugation reactions it is futile to expect to discern the relationship between the fate of foreign compounds and the effects they elicit in biological systems. In addition, a fresh look at the conjugation reactions and their interrelation with intermediary metabolism may serve to open new horizons in biochemistry and pathology.

REFERENCES

1. R. T. Williams, Detoxication Mechanisms, 2nd ed. Chapman & Hall, London, 1959.
2. A. Conti and M. H. Bickel, Drug Metab. Rev. 6:1 (1977).
3. R. L. Smith and R. T. Williams, in Metabolic Conjugation and Metabolic Hydrolysis (W. H. Fishman, ed.), Vol. 1. Academic Press, New York, 1970, p. 1.
4. R. T. Williams, Gut 13:579 (1972).
5. D. J. Jollow, J. J. Kocsis, R. Snyder, and H. Vainio (eds.), Biological Reactive Intermediates. Plenum Press, New York, 1977.
6. A. A. Sinkula and S. H. Yalkowsky, J. Pharm. Sci. 64:181, 1975.
7. R. L. Smith and R. T. Williams, in Glucuronic Acid Free and Combined (G. J. Dutton, ed.). Academic Press, New York, 1966, p. 457.
8. J. Caldwell, in Conjugation Reactions in Drug Biotransformation (A. Aitio, ed.). Elsevier, Amsterdam, 1978, p. 477.

9. J. Caldwell, Life Sci. 24:571 (1979).

10. R. T. Williams, in Biogenesis of Natural Compounds (P. Bernfeld, ed.), 2nd ed. Pergamon Press, Oxford, N.Y., 1967, p. 589.

11. G. J. Dutton and B. Burchell, Progr. Drug Metab. 2:1 (1977).

12. C. C. Porter, B. H. Arison, V. F. Gruber, D. C. Titus, and W. J. A. Van den Heuvel, Drug Metab. Dispos. 3:189 (1975).

13. W. R. Richter, K. O. Alt, W. Dieterle, J. W. Faigle, H. P. Kriemler, H. Mory, and T. Winkler, Helv. Chim. Acta 58:2512 (1975).

14. W. Dieterle, J. W. Faigle, F. Frueh, H. Mory, W. Theobald, K. O. Alt, and W. R. Richter, Arzneim. Forsch. 26:572 (1976).

15. G. J. Wishart, M. T. Campbell, and G. J. Dutton, in Conjugation Reactions in Drug Biotransformation (A. Aitio, ed.). Elsevier, Amsterdam, 1978, p. 179.

16. E. Del Villar, E. Sanchez, A. P. Autor, and T. R. Tephly, Mol. Pharmacol. 2:236 (1975).

17. G. J. Dutton, in Glucuronic Acid Free and Combined (G. J. Dutton, ed.). Academic Press, New York, 1966, p. 186.

18. G. J. Dutton, G. J. Wishart, J. E. A. Leakey, and M. A. Goheer, in Drug Metabolism from Microbe to Man (D. V. Parke and R. L. Smith, eds.). Taylor & Francis, London, 1977, p. 71.

19. H. P. Pan and J. R. Fouts, Drug Metab. Rev. 7:1 (1978).

20. J. N. Smith, in Drug Metabolism from Microbe to Man (D. V. Parke and R. L. Smith, eds.). Taylor & Francis, London, 1977, p. 219.

21. S. M. Sieber and R. H. Adamson, in Drug Metabolism from Microbe to Man (D. V. Parke and R. L. Smith, eds.). Taylor & Francis, London, 1977, p. 233.

22. J. Caldwell, R. T. Williams, M. R. French, and O. Bassir, Eur. J. Drug Metab. 2:61 (1978).

23. B. C. Baldwin, in Drug Metabolism from Microbe to Man (D. V. Parke and R. L. Smith, eds.). Taylor & Francis, London, 1977, p. 191.

24. K. P. M. Heirwegh, in Conjugation Reactions in Drug Biotransformation (A. Aitio, ed.). Elsevier, Amsterdam, 1978, p. 67.

25. D. E. Duggan, J. J. Baldwin, B. H. Arison, and R. E. Rhodes, J. Pharmacol. Exp. Ther. 190:563 (1974).

26. W. Kalow, Abstr. Symp. Multiple Forms of Cytochrome P-450, London, 1978.

27. R. S. Labow and D. S. Layne, Biochem. J. 128:491 (1972).

28. M. A. Schwartz, S. J. Kolis, T. H. Williams, T. F. Gabriel, and V. Toome, Drug Metab. Dispos. 1:557 (1973).

29. H. G. Mandel, Pharmacol. Rev. 11:743 (1959).

30. J. Fevery, M. Van der Vijver, R. Michiels, and K. P. M. Heirwegh, Biochem. J. 164:737 (1977).

31. A. B. Roy, Handb. Exp. Pharmakol. 28(2):536 (1971).

32. G. M. Powell, J. J. Miller, A. H. Olavesen, and C. G. Curtis, Nature 252:234 (1974).

33. J. D. Gregory, Methods Enzymol. $\underline{5}$:982 (1962).
34. K. S. Dodgson, in Drug Metabolism from Microbe to Man (D. V. Parke and R. L. Smith, eds.). Taylor & Francis, London, 1977, p. 91.
35. P. C. Hirom, J. R. Idle, and P. Millburn, in Drug Metabolism from Microbe to Man (D. V. Parke and R. L. Smith, eds.). Taylor & Francis, London, 1977, p. 299.
36. G. Levy, in Conjugation Reactions in Drug Biotransformation (A. Aitio, ed.). Elsevier, Amsterdam, 1978, p. 469.
37. I. D. Capel, M. R. French, P. Millburn, R. L. Smith, and R. T. Williams, Xenobiotica $\underline{2}$:25 (1972).
38. G. Levy and T. Matsuzawa, J. Pharmacol. Exp. Ther. $\underline{156}$:285 (1967).
39. G. J. Mulder and A. B. D. van Doorn, Abstr. 6th Int. Cong. Pharmacol., Helsinki, 1975, No. 292.
40. J. S. Wold, R. L. Smith, and R. T. Williams, Biochem. Pharmacol. $\underline{22}$:1865 (1973).
41. P. Laduron, in Frontiers in Catecholamine Research (E. Usdin and S. H. Snyder, eds.). Pergamon Press, Oxford, 1974, p. 121.
42. S. H. Mudd, in Metabolic Conjugation and Metabolic Hydrolysis (W. H. Fishman, ed.), Vol. 3. Academic Press, New York, 1973, p. 298.
43. W. C. Govier, J. Pharmacol. Exp. Ther. $\underline{150}$:305 (1965).
44. D. E. Drayer and M. M. Reidenberg, Clin. Pharmacol. Ther. $\underline{22}$:251 (1977).
45. W. Kalow, Pharmacogenetics. Saunders, Philadelphia, 1962.
46. W. W. Weber, J. N. Miceli, D. J. Hearse, and G. S. Drummond, Drug Metab. Dispos. $\underline{4}$:94 (1976).
47. J. H. Peters, G. R. Gordon, and P. Brown, Proc. Soc. Exp. Biol. Med. $\underline{120}$:575 (1965).
48. G. J. Dutton, in Drug Metabolism in Man (J. W. Gorrod, ed.). Taylor & Francis, London, 1978, p. 81.
49. J. Caldwell, J. R. Idle, and R. L. Smith, in Extrahepatic Metabolism of Drugs and Other Foreign Compounds (T. E. Gram, ed.). Spectrum Publ., Holliswood, N.Y., 1970, in press.
50. J. Caldwell, in Conjugation Reactions in Drug Biotransformation (A. Aitio, ed.). Elsevier, Amsterdam, 1978, p. 111.
51. D. M. Jerina and J. R. Bend, in Biological Reactive Intermediates (D. J. Jollow, J. J. Kocsis, R. Snyder, and H. Vainio, eds.). Plenum Press, New York, 1977, p. 207.
52. W. H. Habig, J. H. Keengood, and W. B. Jakoby, Biochem. Biophys. Res. Commun. $\underline{64}$:501 (1975).
53. H. Sies, G. Gerstnecker, H. Menzel, and L. Fishe, FEBS Lett. $\underline{27}$:171 (1972).
54. P. L. Grover, in Drug Metabolism from Microbe to Man (D. V. Parke and R. L. Smith, eds.). Taylor & Francis, London, 1977, p. 105.
55. R. L. Smith, The Excretory Function of Bile. Chapman & Hall, London, 1973.

56. R. T. Williams and P. Millburn, in <u>Physiological and Pharmacological</u> <u>Biochemistry</u> (H. K. F. Blaschko, ed.), MTP Int. Rev. Sci., Ser. 1, Vol. 12. Butterworths, London, 1975, p. 211.
57. J. Weinstock, S. E. Parker, G. W. Lucyszyn, and A. P. Intoccia, Pharmacologist 11:240 (1969).
58. E. G. Leighty, A. F. Fentiman, Jr., and R. L. Foltz, Res. Commun. Chem. Pathol. Pharmacol. 14:13 (1976).
59. I. D. Capel, P. Millburn, and R. T. Williams, Biochem. Soc. Trans. 2:305 (1974).
60. D. E. Hathway (ed.), <u>Foreign Compound Metabolism in Mammals</u>, Vol. 1. Chemical Soc., London, 1970, p. 380.
61. W. G. Stilwell, O. J. Bouwsma, G. W. Griffin, and M. G. Horning, Abst. 7th Int. Cong. Pharmacol., Paris, 1978, No. 2579.
62. Z. H. Israili, P. G. Dayton, and J. R. Kiechel, Drug Metab. Dispos. 5:411 (1977).
63. P. Jenner and B. Testa, Xenobiotica 8:1 (1978).
64. <u>Toxic Substances List</u>, 1973 ed. U.S. Dept. of Health, Education, and Welfare, Rockville, Md., 1973.
65. R. T. Williams, Biochem. Soc. Trans. 2:359 (1974).
66. R. Schmid, in <u>Metabolic Basis of Inherited Disease</u> (J. B. Stanbury, J. B. Wyngaarden, and D. S. Fredrickson, eds.), 3rd ed. McGraw-Hill, New York, 1972, p. 1141.
67. M. S. Ebadi and R. B. Kugel, Pediat. Res. 4:187 (1970).
68. C. C. Irving, in <u>Biological Oxidation of Nitrogen</u> (J. W. Gorrod, ed.). Elsevier, Amsterdam, 1978, p. 325.
69. R. T. Williams, Envir. Health Persp. 22:133 (1978).
70. J. R. Mitchell, D. J. Jollow, W. Z. Potter, D. C. Davis, J. R. Gillette, and B. B. Brodie, J. Pharmacol. Exp. Ther. 187:185 (1973).
71. J. R. Mitchell, S. S. Thorgeirsson, W. Z. Potter, and D. J. Jollow, Clin. Pharmacol. Ther. 16:676 (1974).
72. H. J. Kaufman, Deut. Med. Wochenschr. 85:1090 (1960).
73. P. Sims, P. L. Grover, A. Swaisland, K. Pal, and A. Hewer, Nature 252:326 (1974).
74. N. Nemoto and H. V. Gelboin, Biochem. Pharmacol. 25:1221 (1976).
75. N. Nemoto and S. Takayama, Biochem. Pharmacol. 26:679 (1977).
76. J. Caldwell and P. S. Sever, Clin. Pharmacol. Ther. 16:989 (1974).
77. S. Y. Yeh, R. L. McQuinn, and C. W. Gorodetzky, J. Pharmacol. Exp. Ther. 66:201 (1977).
78. R. Schulz and A. Goldstein, J. Pharmacol. Exp. Ther. 183:404 (1972).
79. M. Mori, K. Oguri, H. Yoshimura, K. Shimomura, O. Kamata, and S. Ueki, Life Sci. 11:525 (1972).
80. A. Bulaid, I. M. James, C. M. Kaye, O. R. W. Lewellen, E. Roberts, M. Sankey, J. Smith, R. Templeton, and R. T. Thomas, Brit. J. Clin. Pharmacol. 5:261 (1978).

81. L. L. Iversen, The Uptake and Storage of Noradrenaline in Sympathetic Nerves. Cambridge Univ. Press, Cambridge, 1967.

82. C. T. Dollery, D. S. Davies, and M. E. Conolly, Ann. N.Y. Acad. Sci. 179:108 (1971).

83. M. Mason, in Metabolic Conjugation and Metabolic Hydrolysis (W. H. Fishman, ed.), Vol. 1. Academic Press, New York, 1970, p. 98.

84. J. A. Miller and E. C. Miller, in Biological Reactive Intermediates (D. J. Jollow, J. J. Kocsis, R. Snyder, and H. Vainio, eds.). Plenum Press, New York, 1977, p. 6.

85. C. C. Irving, in Metabolic Conjugation and Metabolic Hydrolysis (W. H. Fishman, ed.), Vol. 1. Academic Press, New York, 1970, p. 53.

86. F. Kadlubar, J. A. Miller, and E. C. Miller, Cancer Res. 37:305 (1977).

87. J. R. Mitchell (moderator), Ann. Intern. Med. 84:181 (1976).

88. I. Sperber, Ann. Roy. Agr. Coll. Sweden 15:317 (1948).

89. I. Sperber, Ann. Roy. Agr. Coll. Sweden 16:49 (1948).

90. G. Levy, T. Tsuchiya, and L. P. Amsel, Clin. Pharmacol. Ther. 13:258 (1972).

91. M. Rowland, in Drug Metabolism from Microbe to Man (D. V. Parke and R. L. Smith, eds.). Taylor & Francis, London, 1977, p. 123.

92. J. G. Wagner, in Pharmacology and Pharmacokinetics (T. Teorell, R. L. Dedrick, and R. G. Condliffe, eds.). Plenum Press, New York, 1974, p. 27.

93. N. Gerber and J. G. Wagner, Res. Commun. Chem. Pathol. Pharmacol. 3:455 (1972).

94. J. Caldwell, R. Lancaster, T. J. Monks, and R. L. Smith, Brit. J. Clin. Pharmacol. 4:637P (1977).

95. F. Lundquist and H. Wolthers, Acta Pharmacol. Toxicol. 14:265 (1958).

96. D. J. Jollow, S. S. Thorgeirsson, W. Z. Potter, M. Hashimoto, and J. R. Mitchell, Pharmacology 12:251 (1974).

97. G. Levy and J. A. Procknal, J. Pharm. Sci. 60:215 (1971).

98. G. Levy and H. Yamada, J. Pharm. Sci. 60:215 (1971).

99. K. Kakemi, T. Arita, H. Sezaki, and M. Hanano, J. Pharm. Soc., Japan 83:260 (1963).

100. M. M. Drucker, S. H. Blondheim, and L. Wislicki, Clin. Sci. 27:133 (1964).

101. G. Levy and K. M. Giacomini, Clin. Pharmacol. Ther. 23:247 (1978).

102. J. Caldwell and R. L. Smith, in Formulation and Preparation of Dosage Forms (J. Polderman, ed.). Elsevier, Amsterdam, 1977, p. 169.

103. R. Minder, F. Schnetzer, and M. H. Bickel, Naunyn-Schmeidebergs Arch. Pharmakol. Exp. Path. 268:334 (1971).

104. A. J. Glazko, W. A. Dill, and L. M. Wolf, J. Pharmacol. Exp. Ther. 104:452 (1952).

105. R. Thomson, M. Sturtevant, O. D. Bird, and A. J. Glazko, Endocrinology 55:665 (1954).
106. H. B. Hucker, A. G. Zacchei, S. V. Cox, D. A. Brodie, and N. H. R. Cantwell, J. Pharmacol. Exp. Ther. 153:237 (1966).
107. R. L. Smith and P. Millburn, Proc. 6th Int. Congr. Pharmacol., Vol. 6, p. 78 (1975).
108. P. A. F. Dixon, J. Caldwell, and R. L. Smith, Biochem. Soc. Trans. 2:879 (1974).
109. P. A. F. Dixon, J. Caldwell, and R. L. Smith, Xenobiotica 7:695 (1977).
110. W. D. Conway, S. M. Singhri, M. Gibaldi, and R. N. Boyes, Xenobiotica 3:813 (1973).
111. M. E. Conolly, D. S. Davies, C. T. Dollery, C. D. Morgan, J. W. Paterson, and M. Sandler, Brit. J. Pharmacol. 46:458 (1972).
112. S. Riegelman and M. Rowland, J. Pharmacokin. Biopharm. 5:419 (1973).
113. M. Gibaldi and D. Perrier, Drug Metab. Rev. 3:185 (1974).
114. P. N. Bennett, E. Blackwell, and D. S. Davies, Nature 258:247 (1975).
115. D. J. Jollow and C. Smith, in Biological Reactive Intermediates (D. J. Jollow, J. J. Kocsis, R. Snyder, and H. Vainio, eds.). Plenum Press, New York, 1977, p. 43.
116. I. C. Calder, K. Healey, A. C. Yong, C. A. Crowe, K. N. Ham, and J. D. Tange, in Biological Oxidation of Nitrogen (J. W. Gorrod, ed.). Elsevier, Amsterdam, 1978, p. 309.
117. M. M. Reidenberg and D. E. Drayer, Abstr. 7th Int. Congr. Pharmacol., Paris, 1978, No. 550.

Chapter 5

ROLE OF EXTRAHEPATIC METABOLISM

Harri Vainio

Department of Industrial Hygiene
and Toxicology
Institute of Occupational Health
Helsinki, Finland

Eino Hietanen[*]

Department of Physiology
University of Kuopio
Kuopio, Finland

During the development of sensitive methods for estimating drug-metabolizing enzyme activities numerous extrahepatic organs have been found to be at least slightly active. The liver, however, is a poor predictor of whether a given compound will undergo extrahepatic metabolism. This leads to important implications with respect to drug disposition and tissue-specific activation or detoxication of foreign compounds. Among the most active extrahepatic organs are those related to the entrance or excretion of xenobiotics to or from the body, including skin, gastrointestinal tract, lungs, and kidneys. The significance of biotransformation in extrahepatic tissues gains importance in terms of activation of environmental xenobiotics as a possible cause of tissue damage at these sites of entry or excretion, or in more remote tissues. When assessing the fate of compounds in the body, the possibility of both activation and inactivation should be considered and the relative contributions of enzyme systems to both processes should be taken into account. Foreign compounds entering the body with the air or food or through the skin may affect the balance between the activating and inactivating enzyme complexes, giving rise to either harmful or desirable effects. Exposure to naturally occurring enzyme inducers in the diet, and possibly also occupational exposure, may cause a marked induction in specific extrahepatic tissues (e.g., gastrointestinal tract or lungs) such as to affect the disposition of therapeutic drugs.

---

[*]Present affiliation: Department of Physiology, University of Turku, Turku
Finland

251

I. THE SCOPE OF EXTRAHEPATIC DRUG METABOLISM

Although the liver has long been acknowledged as the major site of drug metabolism, many recent studies have emphasized the importance of extrahepatic tissues in the biotransformation of xenobiotics. Even though extrahepatic drug metabolism may not be particularly important in all phases of disposition, it can markedly modify the biological fate and effects of drugs. Extrahepatic drug metabolism is also of paramount importance in regulating the fate of foreign compounds other than drugs, for example, environmental pollutants in air and water, food additives and contaminants, industrial chemicals, or cigarette smoke. Since the drug-metabolizing enzyme system is also able to activate or inactivate chemicals that are primary or secondary carcinogens, and since 90% of all cancers may be of environmental origin, extrahepatic biotransformation has received increasing attention [1-3].

The sites of extrahepatic drug metabolism are often the portals of entry or excretion of the body, e.g., the lung, kidney, skin, and gastrointestinal mucosa. Thus, extrahepatic metabolism converts foreign compounds to either active or inactive forms preceding their entry into the circulatory system and access to the target tissue. The rate of extrahepatic metabolism may not be as high as in liver and the total capacity may also be lower, but human exposure to both environmental and occupational foreign compounds is often a chronic situation in which only small quantities at a time enter the body.

Besides this role in activating or inactivating xenobiotics, extrahepatic drug metabolism may also play a role in excretion. Indeed, the absorption of drugs into the body is influenced by their lipid solubility, whereas their excretion is facilitated by polarity. Although the liver is the major site for the production of drug metabolites, it is possible that, for example, the intestinal mucosa may produce conjugates of absorbed compounds which are excreted back to the intestinal lumen and therefore never reach the circulatory system [4].

The total capacity of an organ to metabolize xenobiotics is biologically much more important than the specific activity per se. Although specific activity may prove to be biochemically more informative than the total activity of the whole organ, physiologically the latter provides a better idea of the function of the organ. Unfortunately only a few studies have compared biotransformation in whole organs with its biological significance. Since the relative organ weights are not constant between species, it is difficult to compare enzyme activities in this manner. To pursue this aim we have tried in this chapter to extrapolate enzyme activities on a whole organ basis, although we have also compared specific activities, since this is the usual way to express data.

A systematic survey of functionalization (Phase I) reactions [5-12], microsomal enzymes [13-17], and conjugation (Phase II) reactions [18-21] is outside the scope of this chapter. To help the reader, however, a functional scheme of important reactions and enzymes to be considered in this chapter is presented in Fig. 1.

II. TISSUE DISTRIBUTION OF DRUG-METABOLIZING ENZYMES

A. The Drug-Metabolizing Enzymes in Various Extrahepatic Organs

1. Functionalization reactions

a. Cytochrome P-450: Table 1 illustrates the distribution of cytochrome P-450 in tissues of various species [5, 22-45]. Thus, rat liver contains about 0.55 nmol/mg protein, which is equivalent to 12.3 nmol/g wet weight, the calculated total amount in liver being 123 nmol (Table 2). In a similar way, intestinal activity can be extrapolated if it is assumed that the activity remains the same in the whole length of the small intestine (which does not happen). If the average weight of rat small intestine is about 3 g, the maximal total cytochrome P-450 content can be estimated to be about 2 nmol. In the rat the total intestinal cytochrome P-450 is about 1.6% of the level in the liver (Table 2). In the rat kidney, there is approximately 3.5 nmol of cytochrome P-450 present since the average organ weight is 2.1 g, the microsomal protein concentration is 10 mg/g wet weight, and the cytochrome content is 0.16 nmol/mg protein.

The data in Table 1 indicate the marked interspecies variation in cytochrome P-450 levels. In contrast to the rat, rabbit intestinal and renal cytochrome P-450 contents per milligram of microsomal protein are nearly one-third of that in the liver. The species differences that exist are further illustrated by pulmonary cytochrome P-450 levels, which vary from 0.035 to 0.38 nmol/mg, depending on the species. In rats, pulmonary cytochrome

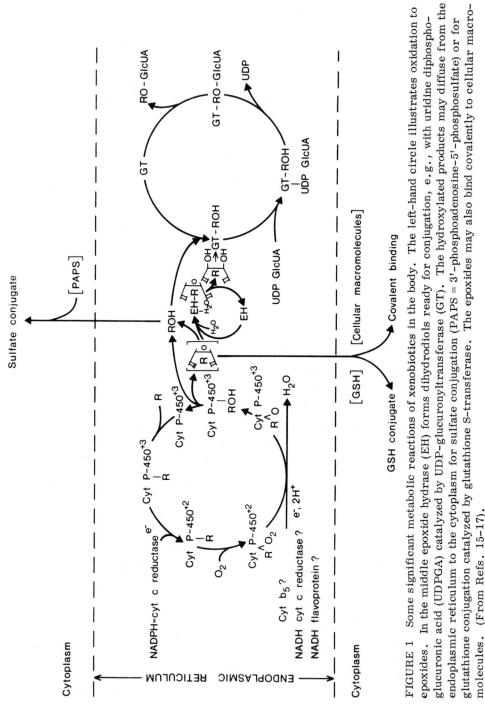

FIGURE 1 Some significant metabolic reactions of xenobiotics in the body. The left-hand circle illustrates oxidation to epoxides. In the middle epoxide hydrase (EH) forms dihydrodiols ready for conjugation, e.g., with uridine diphosphoglucuronic acid (UDPGA) catalyzed by UDP-glucuronyltransferase (GT). The hydroxylated products may diffuse from the endoplasmic reticulum to the cytoplasm for sulfate conjugation (PAPS = 3'-phosphoadenosine-5'-phosphosulfate) or for glutathione conjugation catalyzed by glutathione S-transferase. The epoxides may also bind covalently to cellular macromolecules. (From Refs. 15-17).

TABLE 1
Cytochrome P-450 in Various Tissues

Organ	Species				
	Rat	Mouse	Rabbit	Guinea pig	Human
Liver	0.22-0.92	0.39-1.10	0.81-1.70	0.43-1.45	0.26-1.02
Kidney	0.05-0.21	0.40	0.14-0.36	0.32	0.030
Lung	0.035	--	0.27-0.38	0.07	--
Intestine	0.01-0.13	0.04	0.07-0.43	0.18	--
Adrenal gland	0.50	--	1.20	2.0	0.23-0.54
Testis	0.05-0.10	0.24	0.040	0.078	0.005
Skin	0.05	0.022	--	--	--
Spleen	0.025	--	--	--	--
Ovary	--	--	0.06	--	--
Brain	0.025-0.051	--	--	--	--

[a] nmol/mg microsomal protein.
Source: Data from Refs. 5 and 22-45.

TABLE 2
Organ Distribution of the Drug-Metabolizing Enzymes in the Rat[a]

Enzyme	Liver	Kidneys	Lungs	Intestinal mucosa	Adrenal gland	Spleen	Brain
Cytochrome P-450							
nmol/mg protein	0.55	0.16	0.035	0.13	0.50	0.025	0.036
nmol/organ	122.5	3.5	0.42	1.95	0.18	0.45	0.29
NADPH-cytochrome c reductase							
nmol/mg/protein/min	135	29	55	88	--	--	39
μmol/organ/min	33.8	0.46	0.66	1.32	--	--	0.31

Aryl hydrocarbon hydroxylase							
pmol/g (wet wt)/min	1500	100	300	75	2330	23	0.4
nmol/organ/min	15	0.22	0.36	0.23	0.08	0.03	0.00064
UDP-glucuronyltransferase (methylumbelliferone)							
nmol/g (wet wt)/min	456	145	27	259	174	30	0.8
μmol/organ/min	4.56	0.32	0.032	0.78	0.006	0.009	0.001
Epoxide hydrase (benzpyrene 4,5-oxide)							
pmol/mg protein/min	6391	705	362	126	259	140	104
nmol/organ/min	1598	15.5	4.3	1.9	0.09	2.5	0.8
Estimated organ weight (g)	10	2.2	1.2	3	0.036	1.2	1.6

[a] The specific concentration or activities are approximate means from Tables 1 and 3.

P-450 is only about 0.34% of the liver levels. The cytochrome P-450 levels in adrenal glands are high in all species (due to its importance in steroidogenesis), but the total amount remains low because of the small size of the organ. Other endocrine organs such as testes and ovaries have cytochrome P-450 levels comparable to those in intestine and lungs (Table 1). Skin and brain also contain some microsomal cytochrome P-450.

b. NADPH-cytochrome c reductase: The specific NADPH-cytochrome c reductase activity in rat liver is 135 nmol/mg microsomal protein/minute, which yields 34 μmol/liver/minute (Tables 2 and 3). In rat intestine, however, the specific activity varies from 42.2 to 133.8 nmol/mg microsomal protein/minute, which results in a total intestinal activity of some 0.6-2.0 μmol/small intestine/minute, or 3% of hepatic activity. Similarly, the renal activity varies from 6.4 to 52 nmol/mg microsomal protein/minute, which gives 0.12-1.1 μmol of reduced cytochrome c/two kidneys/minute in rats. In rabbits and guinea pigs the distribution is similar to that found in rats. The cytochrome c reductase activity of almost all tissues including brain therefore appears to be rather high [16,24,28,31, 37,39,40,42-44,46-51].

c. Aryl hydrocarbon hydroxylase: The specific aryl hydrocarbon hydroxylase activity in subcellular fractions of the rat intestine varies from 5 to 40% of the respective liver activities (Table 4), whereas the total intestinal activity varies from 1.5 to 10% of the liver levels (Table 2). Similarly, rabbit intestinal aryl hydrocarbon hydroxylase activity is about 10% of the respective hepatic activity (Table 4). In contrast, mouse intestinal aryl hydrocarbon hydroxylase activity varies from 0.6 to 68% of hepatic specific activity. Renal activities are in the same range as intestinal activity, whereas the aryl hydrocarbon hydroxylase activity found in the adrenal glands of rats is comparable to the hepatic levels. Aryl hydrocarbon hydroxylase activity has in addition been found in the ovaries, spleen, and pancreas. (See references cited in Table 4.) Juchau et al. [58] have also detected such activity in the walls of blood vessels in monkeys and humans. Marked species variation is apparent in aryl hydrocarbon hydroxylase activity, but an assessment of the true enzyme distribution is partially hampered by large interlaboratory variations [63].

d. Ethoxycoumarin O-deethylase: Examination of the distribution of specific ethoxycoumarin O-deethylase activity in different tissues in rats, mice, and guinea pigs showed that most activity occurred in the liver in all species, although kidneys, lungs, intestinal mucosa, adrenal glands, and spleen also displayed considerable activity (Table 5) [70]. Ullrich [71], when comparing the whole-organ activity of ethoxycoumarin deethylase, found that the liver was responsible for 86.5% of the total activity of mice, while the intestinal mucosa accounted for 8.5%, the skin 4%, the lungs 1%, the kidneys 0.1%, and the brain and heart 0.01% each.

TABLE 3
Organ Distribution of NADPH-Cytochrome c Reductase Activity[a] in Various Species

Species	Liver	Kidney	Lung	Intestine	Skin	Brain
Rat	101–187	6.4–52	55	42.4–133.8	––	26–55
Mouse	109–113	77	133	90	7.9	––
Rabbit	90–238	19–34	58–94	72–140	––	––
Guinea pig	55–225	57	93	44	––	––
Human	61–78	8.2–12	––	––	––	––

[a] nmol/mg microsomal protein/min.
Source: Data from Refs. 16, 24, 28, 31, 37, 39, 40, 42–44, and 46–51.

TABLE 4
Activity of Aryl Hydrocarbon Hydroxylase (nmol/min) in Various Species

Organ	Rat	Mouse	Rabbit	Guinea pig	Monkey	Human
			Species			
Liver						
per mg protein	0.04–0.58	0.22	0.1–1.26	2.9	0.249	0.01
per g (wet wt)	0.21–2.1	2.5	–	–	–	0.24
Kidney						
per mg protein	0.005–0.04	0.0002	0.005–0.015	–	0.003	–
per g (wet wt)	0.004–0.37	0.03	–	–	–	–
Lung						
per mg protein	0.005	0.003	0.015	–	0.015	–
per g (wet wt)	0.13–0.49	0.02–0.2	–	–	–	–
Pancreas						
per mg protein	–	–	0.002	0.0015	–	–

	1	2	3	4	5	6
Intestine						
per mg protein	0.0003–0.09	—	0.05–0.07	—	—	—
per g (wet wt)	0.05–7.3	0.016–1.7	0.14	0.29–0.32	—	—
Mammary gland						
per mg protein	—	0.0001	—	—	0.115	—
Adrenal gland						
per mg protein	—	—	0.050	—	—	—
per g (wet wt)	2.33	—	—	—	—	—
Brain						
per mg protein	0.00008	—	—	—	—	—
Skin						
per mg protein	0.004	0.007–0.017	—	0.0004	—	0.0001
per g (wet wt)	0.001–0.033	0.67	—	—	—	—
Spleen						
per mg protein	0.0165	—	—	—	0.116	—
Ovary						
per mg protein	—	0.00097–0.00157	—	—	—	—

Source: Data from Refs. 18, 22, 27, 29, 31, 32, 39, 40, 42, and 51–59.

TABLE 5
Relative Ethoxycoumarin O-Deethylase Activity in
Various Organs of Guinea Pigs, Rats, and Mice

Organ	Guinea pig	Rat	Mouse
Liver	100[a]	100	100
Kidney	0.7	2.0	6.7
Lung	12.6	5.8	2.8
Testis	0.3	0.5	0.8
Spleen	0.3	0.6	0.2
Adrenal gland	5.3	5.8	5.0
Duodenum	3.6	2.4	3.8

[a]Liver specific activity is denoted by 100.
Source: From Ref. 70.

e. Epoxide hydrase: The distribution of epoxide hydrase using styrene oxide as substrate has been investigated in rats and rabbits (Table 6)
[72,73]. Specific epoxide hydrase activity in the small intestinal mucosa
of the rat was 5% of hepatic activity. This low activity is reflected in the
accumulation of the 4,5-epoxide in incubations of benzo[a]pyrene [39]. In
the rabbit, however, the intestinal epoxide hydrase activity is up to 40% of
the hepatic level when expressed per milligram of microsomal protein
(Table 6). In rabbit kidney, the activity is 25% of the hepatic level, but in
guinea pig kidney it is 8% of hepatic activity [72,73]. Several studies have
calculated the whole-organ activity of epoxide hydrase. Thus, the intestinal
mucosa of rabbit was found to have an epoxide hydrase capacity of 0.39
μmol/min, whereas in the kidney the whole organ capacity was 0.36 μmol/
min and in the liver 11.3 μmol/min [72]. Therefore intestinal capacity was
3% of hepatic capacity, and renal activity was in the same range as intestinal activity. In Table 6 the marked variation in the organ distribution of
epoxide hydrase between rat and rabbit can be seen. This work was confirmed by Oesch and colleagues [74], who studied epoxide hydrase distribution in rats using benzpyrene 4,5-oxide as the substrate (Table 6). Their
organ distribution agreed essentially with the one determined by James et
al. [72,73]. Oesch and co-workers [74] also found marked epoxide hydrase
activity in the spleen, adrenal glands, and brain, as well as in those tissues
related to the entry or excretion of xenobiotics.

TABLE 6
Organ Distribution of Epoxide Hydrase in the Rat and Rabbit

	Rat		Rabbit	
Organ	nmol/mg protein/ min	μmol/organ/ min	nmol/mg protein/ min	μmol/organ/ min
Liver	4.9-6.8	1.23	5.6	11.3
Kidneys	0.58-0.76	0.013	1.4	0.36
Lungs	0.46	--	0.17	0.02
Intestine	0.1-0.23	0.0015-0.0035	2.8	0.39

Source: Data from Refs. 65, 72, and 73.

2. Conjugation reactions

a. Glutathione S-transferase: In the small intestinal mucosa of rats the glutathione S-transferase activity per milligram of cytoplasmic protein is 9% of the hepatic activity (Table 7). In the rabbit the intestinal activity is 14% of the hepatic level, and in the guinea pig 10%. The renal activity, on the other hand, is 26% of the hepatic activity in rabbits but only 3% in the guinea pig. Rats in contrast have an exceptionally high specific renal gluta-thione S-transferase activity, which is 60% of the hepatic activity (Table 7), although the whole-organ activity is only 4.5% of total hepatic activity. In the rabbit the whole-intestinal glutathione S-transferase activity is 1% of the hepatic whole-organ activity, and the renal whole-organ activity is about 1.5% of that in the liver. In rats the intestinal activity is only 0.5% of the whole hepatic glutathione S-transferase level (Table 7). It must be noted, however, that in rats and guinea pigs the hepatic specific activity is much higher than in rabbits.

b. UDP-glucuronyltransferase: UDP-glucuronyltransferase(s) cata-lyzes the conjugation of xenobiotics and endogenous compounds with glu-curonic acid. The tissue distribution of UDP-glucuronyltransferase activity varies depending on the substrate used. With 4-methylumbelliferone as the substrate, the organ distribution of UDP-glucuronyltransferase activity in rats has been studied by Aitio [18]. The results show the activity (per gram

TABLE 7

Glutathione S-Transferase[a] Activity in Various Tissues
of the Rat, Rabbit, and Guinea Pig

Tissue	Rat		Rabbit		Guinea pig
	nmol/mg protein/ min	μmol/organ/ min	nmol/mg protein/ min	μmol/organ/ min	nmol/mg protein/ min
Liver	141.8	35.5	30.5	240.3	236.5
Kidneys	82.1	1.6	7.9	3.5	7.5
Lung	12.2	0.07	6.5	3.1	18.6
Intestine	12.8	0.19	4.4	2.5	24.6

[a] Here, [^{14}C]styrene oxide is the substrate.
Source: Data from Refs. 72 and 73.

of tissue wet weight) in the duodenum to be about 57% of that in the liver.
The adrenal, renal, and pulmonary and splenic activities were found to be
37, 32, and 6%, respectively, of the hepatic specific activity. A slight activity was even found in the brain (Table 2). All activity was measured using
a digitonin-activated 9000g supernatant as the enzyme source. Due to the
latency of UDP-glucuronyltransferase, maximal activity is seen only after
various in vitro membrane treatments. The in vivo activity may thus be
quite different from that measured in vitro. Keeping these facts in mind, it
is nevertheless feasible to extrapolate UDP-glucuronyltransferase activites
on a whole-organ basis (Table 2). Based on these assumptions, the intestinal mucosa has 17% of the total hepatic UDP-glucuronyltransferase activity
while the renal capacity is 7% and pulmonary 0.7% of the hepatic capacity.
However, when para-nitrophenol is used as the substrate [75], the intestinal mucosa has apparently twice the activity found in the liver per gram
of wet weight. Similarly activity in the kidneys is about 50% higher than in
the liver in digitonin-activated tissue preparations. When ortho-aminophenol is used as the substrate, the duodenal and hepatic activities per
milligram of tissue dry weight are about equal, and renal activity is 30% of
the hepatic activity [76]. The fact that comparisons are not always made
using the same tissue preparations creates some confusion. For further
details on this subject as well as on other conjugation reactions, the recent

review by Aitio and Marniemi [19] on extrahepatic conjugation reactions may be consulted.

B. Classical Enzyme Inducers and Extrahepatic
    Drug Metabolism

Table 8 presents a summary of the induction of cytochrome P-450, ethoxycoumarin O-deethylase, aryl hydrocarbon hydroxylase, epoxide hydrase and UDP-glucuronyltransferase enzymes in rats, guinea pigs, and rabbits by phenobarbital, 3-methylcholanthrene, and 2,3,7,8-tetrachlorodibenzopara-dioxin (TCDD). The response to induction varies in different tissues [22,23,29,32,39,40,47,77,78]. For example, in rat liver and kidney the specific cytochrome P-450 concentration is doubled by phenobarbital treatment, and a similar hepatic response occurs in the rabbit and guinea pig. Intestinal cytochrome P-450, on the other hand, is highly inducible in rats, but in the small intestine of rabbits only slight induction takes place. In rabbit kidney TCDD, phenobarbital, and 3-methylcholanthrene are potent inducers of aryl hydrocarbon hydroxylase activity. The lungs, in contrast, appear nonresponsive to phenobarbital and 3-methylcholanthrene, while TCDD induces both aryl hydrocarbon hydroxylase and UDP-glucuronyltransferase activities in this tissue.

The different responses of the monooxygenase system to enzyme inducers in various species and tissues may be due to the existence of multiple forms of cytochrome P-450. Zampaglione and Mannering [69], for example, have suggested the existence of two aryl hydrocarbon hydroxylase enzymes in the liver—one utilizing cytochrome P-450 as terminal oxidase; and the other, cytochrome P-448. In contrast, a P-448-dependent aryl hydrocarbon hydroxylase predominates in the intestinal mucosa of both untreated and 3-methylcholanthrene-induced rats. Adrenal aryl hydrocarbon hydroxylase is different from that of the liver and intestinal mucosa and is not inducible by 3-methylcholanthrene. It seems that a cytochrome P-448-dependent aryl hydrocarbon hydroxylase exists in such portals of entry of xenobiotics as the intestine, skin, and lungs. These results are important because they indicate that the differences between the monooxygenase systems of the liver and extrahepatic organs are not only quantitative but also qualitative in nature.

Inspection of Table 9 [77] indicates a two- to tenfold induction of aryl hydrocarbon hydroxylase by benzo[a]pyrene in extrahepatic tissues of rats. Other inducers also display considerable activity. Thus, Iqbal and collaborators have shown guinea pig pancreatic aryl hydrocarbon hydroxylase activity to be induced approximately 15-fold by 3-methylcholanthrene [57]. In rat skin, a single application of polychlorinated biphenyls induces aryl hydrocarbon hydroxylase 25- to 40-fold [53]. Various polycyclic aromatic hydrocarbons and benzoflavones are also potent inducers of cutaneous aryl hydrocarbon hydroxylase, the highest enzymic activity being found in the

TABLE 8
Extrahepatic Enzyme Induction[a]

Organ	Cytochrome P-450 (nmol/mg)	Ethoxycoumarin O-deethylase (nmol/mg/min)	Aryl hydrocarbon hydroxylase (pmol/mg/min)	Epoxide hydrase (pmol styrene glycol/mg/min)	UDP-glucuronyltransferase (pNP)[b] (nmol/mg/min)
RAT					
Liver:					
Control	0.85-1.41	0.400	390-580	13.5	30.4
PB[c]	1.95-2.55	1.32	340	55.7	--
3MC[d]	1.12-2.46	--	2660	--	--
TCDD[e]	--	--	1480	--	154.9
Lungs:					
Control	0.23	--	<10	--	0.55
PB	0.24	--	--	--	--
3MC	0.30	--	--	--	--
TCDD	--	--	40	--	3.12
Kidneys:					
Control	0.15	--	<10	--	8.18
PB	0.33	--	--	--	--
3MC	0.27	--	--	--	--
TCDD	--	--	770	--	44.22
Gut:					
Control	0.02	0.11	80	--	0.95
PB	0.11	0.20	150	--	--
3MC	0.11	1.91	2100	--	--
TCDD	--	--	180	--	3.45

GUINEA PIG

Liver:					
Control	0.93	0.76	155	56.0	62.4
PB	1.60	4.34	252	79.0	--
3MC	--	--	--	--	--
TCDD	--	--	--	--	74.9
Lungs:					
Control	0.18	0.29	19	1.7	0.89
PB	0.13	0.31	14	1.5	--
3MC	--	--	--	--	--
TCDD	--	--	--	--	1.15
Kidneys:					
Control	--	--	<10	--	8.71
PB	--	--	--	--	--
3MC	--	--	--	--	--
TCDD	--	--	70	--	6.80
Gut:					
Control	0.13	0.13	15	15.0	--
PB	0.20	0.34	24	15.0	--
3MC	--	--	--	--	--
TCDD	--	--	--	--	--

TABLE 8 (continued)

Organ	Cytochrome P-450 (nmol/mg)	Ethoxycoumarin O-Deethylase (nmol/mg/min)	Aryl hydrocarbon hydroxylase (pmol/mg/min)	Epoxide hydrase (pmol styrene glycol/mg/min)	UDP-glucuronyltransferase (pNP)[b] (nmol/mg/min)
RABBIT					
Liver:					
Control	0.81-1.52	2.27	97	--	36.0
PB	2.60-2.66	2.93	450	--	--
3MC	2.05-3.58	0.92	100	--	--
TCDD	2.34	1.13	110	--	38.8
Lungs:					
Control	0.40	--	--	--	0.87
PB	0.38	--	--	--	--
3MC	0.40	--	--	--	--
TCDD	--	--	--	--	1.29
Kidneys:					
Control	--	<0.010	4.7	--	4.72
PB	--	0.029	15	--	--
3MC	--	0.079	26	--	--
TCDD	--	0.066	13	--	3.90
Gut:					
Control	0.34	--	--	--	--
PB	0.32	--	--	--	--
3MC	0.47	--	--	--	--
TCDD	--	--	--	--	--

[a] All activities are given on microsomal protein basis.
[b] pNP, para-Nitrophenol.
[c] PB, Phenobarbital.
[d] 3MC, 3-Methylcholanthrene.
[e] TCDD, 2,3,7,8-Tetrachlorodibenzo-para-dioxin.
Source: Data from Refs. 22, 23, 29, 32, 39, 40, 47, 77, and 78.

TABLE 9
Aryl Hydrocarbon Hydroxylase[a] Induction in
Extrahepatic Tissues by Benzo[a]pyrene

Organ	Control	Benzo[a]pyrene
Lymph node	0.0032	0.0349
Lung	0.0265	0.273
Prostate	0.0095	0.0492
Kidney	0.193	0.714
Salivary gland	0.0053	0.0145
Liver	3.19	7.268
Spleen	0.0165	0.033
Mammary gland	0.0046	0.0423

[a] pmol OH-BP/mg (wet weight)/min.
Source: From Ref. 77.

superficial layer of the skin, while activities are intermediate in the epi-
dermis and lowest in the deeper dermal layers [68; see also 68a]. Taken
globally, these results suggest a considerable potential capacity of extrahepatic organs for biotransformation. Recognition of this capacity and its
pharmacological and toxicological implications is rather recent but is becoming rapidly widespread.

The route of administration is also important in the regulation of induction, especially where the lungs and intestine are concerned. Thus,
intestinal aryl hydrocarbon hydroxylase is inducible by intragastric doses
of benzo[a]pyrene so low as not to cause induction after intraperitoneal
administration [29].

The differences between hepatic and extrahepatic tissues in responding
to inducers are reflected in the metabolic patterns of test substances. Thus,
the metabolites of benzo[a]pyrene (BP) in control and 3-methylcholanthrene-
induced intestinal microsomes are similar, but they differ markedly from
the hepatic metabolites [38,80]. Major intestinal metabolites are quinones,
the 4,5-oxide, and the 3- and 9-hydroxy-BP. Only small amounts of dihydrodiols were detected, in contrast to the findings in the liver; this fact,
together with the accumulation of the 4,5-oxide, suggests a low epoxide
hydrase activity in the intestinal mucosa. 3-Methylcholanthrene causes a
maximal induction of about fivefold in the intestinal cytochrome P-450 concentrations, while amounts of benzo[a]pyrene metabolites are increased
about 30-fold, as is aryl hydrocarbon hydroxylase activity. As a consequence,

the intestinal mucosa in the induced state may have as high a monooxygenase activity as the induced liver on a milligram of protein basis.

To summarize this section, it appears that several organs may display
after induction a specific biotransformation as high as that of the induced
liver. Moreover, due to qualitative differences between hepatic and extrahepatic monooxygenase systems, some chemicals and drugs may be prone
to be better substrates for the latter than for the former systems. The
qualitative and quantitative differences seen between the liver and other
organs in some metabolic pathways make the fate of xenobiotics in animals
and humans even more complex, and hence make it imperative for us to gain
a global understanding of drug metabolism at the whole-body level.

III. MODIFIERS OF DRUG METABOLISM IN
     EXTRAHEPATIC TISSUES

A. Nutrition

The effects of nutrition on biotransformation have been studied through the
provision of diets either deficient in some component(s) or purified and for-
tified with a given nutrient(s). In two review articles [81,82], nutritional
influences on drug metabolism have been surveyed; however, these two articles are limited to the liver, despite the fact that the gastrointestinal tract
is the site of entry of nutrients and of many xenobiotics.

Many natural compounds present in foods (e.g., flavones, β-ionone,
safrole, xanthines, indoles) are known to influence drug metabolism (Table
10) [28,65,83-91]. Thus, inducers in plants of the Brassicaceae family
stimulate intestinal phenacetin metabolism three- to sevenfold, while aryl
hydrocarbon hydroxylase activity is stimulated up to 85-fold and ethoxycoumarin O-deethylase activity 43-fold (Table 10). In humans, charcoal-
broiled beef decreased the phenacetin concentration in serum to one-third
of the level measured with the control diet [90]. In agreement, animal
studies showed a 12-fold increase in intestinal phenacetin metabolism after
the consumption of charcoal-broiled meat (Table 10).

Such elementary diet components as iron and cholesterol are able to
modify intestinal drug metabolism. Hoensch and colleagues, for example,
found dietary iron to be essential to the maintenance of the intestinal cytochrome P-450 levels in rats [28]. Dietary cholesterol (2%) is able to stimulate aryl hydrocarbon hydroxylase activity 80-fold in rat intestinal mucosa
(Table 10), and UDP-glucuronyltransferase twofold [85].

These dietary experiments clearly demonstrate that, despite low
"basal" intestinal biotransformation activity, the diet may stimulate enzyme
activities to a degree capable of influencing the plasma levels of drugs.

TABLE 10
Stimulation of Intestinal Drug Metabolism by Nutritional
and Environmental Compounds in the Rat

Diet/compound supplement	Phenacetin metabolism	Ethoxycoumarin O-deethylase	Aryl hydrocarbon hydroxylase
Conventional[a]	1	1	1
Cabbage	3.7	9.6-15.8	11.7-32.9
Brussel sprouts	2.9-6.6	20.0-42.7	28.4-85.5
Cholesterol	--	--	70
Indoles	--	--	11-30
Charcoal-broiled beef	11.8	--	--
Cigarette smoke	1.95	--	3.9-8

[a]Control activity is indicated by 1.
Source: Data from Refs. 28, 65, and 83-91.

B. Environmental Pollution and Smoking

Conney and his coworkers [83,84,86,88,89] have recently reviewed the
regulation of xenobiotic biotransformation by environmental agents and diet
both in man and in experimental animals. Environmental agents may enter
the body either via the gastrointestinal tract or the lungs, although some
resorption also takes place through the skin. Nonoccupational pollution
originates mainly from the air, water, or food; responsible components
include numerous chemicals from polycyclic hydrocarbons to heavy metals
and nitroso compounds.
     Tobacco smoke contains a multitude of substances; to date up to 1150
different chemicals have been identified [92]. They include polycyclic aromatic hydrocarbons, amines, nitriles, alkaloids, phenols, and pesticides.
More than 500 polycyclic aromatic compounds have been found in cigarette
smoke condensates, including benzo[a]pyrene which is presently considered
as the quantitatively most important carcinogenic aromatic hydrocarbon in
cigarette smoke. In addition to their connection with cancer, the various
mutagenic chemicals in cigarette smoke may also play a role in the etiology
of cardiovascular diseases [58].

Cigarette smoke exposure increases aryl hydrocarbon hydroxylase activity in microsomes and homogenates of rat [93,94], hamster [95], and mouse lung [96,97,98] as well as in human alveolar macrophages [99]. When pregnant women smoke, the aryl hydrocarbon hydroxylase activity increases in the placenta [61,100,101]. Similarly, exposing pregnant rats to cigarette smoke increases aryl hydrocarbon hydroxylase activity in the placenta as well as in both maternal and fetal liver [94]. Aryl hydrocarbon hydroxylase activity has also been found to increase in the lung, kidney, and small intestinal mucosa of rats after single or repeated exposure to cigarette smoke (Table 10). These results are consistent with the enhanced covalent binding of intratracheally instilled [^{3}H]benzo[a]pyrene in rats exposed to cigarette smoke or treated with 3-methylcholanthrene [102,103].

Benzo[a]pyrene is also known to be metabolized by human lung [104] and trachea [105], and some of its metabolites are known to be bound covalently to the DNA of human bronchial mucosa [56,106,107]. The in situ metabolism of benzo[a]pyrene in extrahepatic tissues may be critical to its possible carcinogenicity in these tissues.

Cigarette smoking has been shown to stimulate the metabolism of phenacetin in humans [88], and lower plasma concentrations of the drug have been observed in cigarette smokers as compared to nonsmokers. Stimulation of intestinal phenacetin O-dealkylase activity also occurs in rats exposed to cigarette smoke [94]. The stimulatory effect of cigarette smoking on the metabolism of phenacetin and other drugs in the gastrointestinal tract and/or an additional first-pass increase in liver metabolism may explain the lower plasma levels of drugs seen in smokers (Table 10) [88,108-110].

IV. ACTIVATION OF XENOBIOTICS AS A CAUSATIVE MECHANISM FOR EXTRAHEPATIC TISSUE DAMAGE

The concept that detoxication is the inevitable result of xenobiotic biotransformation by mammalian enzymes has undergone modification since it was first described. It has become increasingly apparent in recent years that not only do many metabolites of drugs and other chemicals display biological activity but in many instances these metabolites cause a variety of toxic effects (Fig. 2). In many cases, innocuous chemicals are activated by metabolism in the liver and/or other organs to form highly toxic derivatives. In addition, metabolic conversion can also be carried out by intestinal flora [111,112]; intestinal microbes are even able to produce mutagens from compounds which are nonmutagenic in tests utilizing liver microsomes [111].

The importance of metabolic activation in carcinogenesis has often been demonstrated. Aflatoxins and nitrosamines are probably activated in one stage, aromatic amines in two stages, and polycyclic aromatic hydrocarbons in three stages—to highly active, electrophilic intermediates.

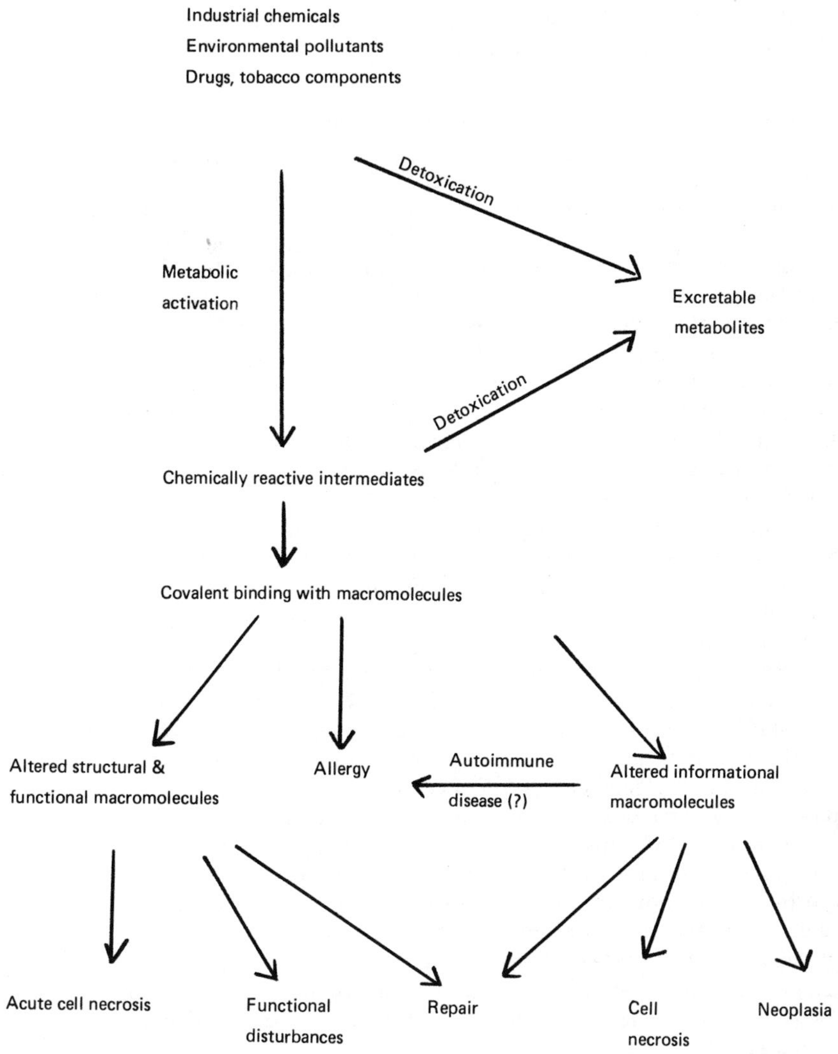

Industrial chemicals

Environmental pollutants

Drugs, tobacco components

FIGURE 2   Formation of active products from xenobiotics and mechanisms of toxicity.

Much of the available information has been obtained with liver and, less frequently, with kidney, gastrointestinal tract, lung and skin preparations. The fact that inactive "precarcinogens" have to be converted into reactive entities indicates that the distribution of induced tumors may depend on metabolic activation. In its final stages at least, this activation may take place locally in specific tissues.

A. Activation of Polycyclic Aromatic Hydrocarbons

Aryl hydrocarbon hydroxylase is present in a variety of tissues of many mammalian species including humans, and it may be induced (see Table 4). The basal and inducible levels vary between tissues as well as between species (see Table 8). There is evidence to believe that aryl hydrocarbon hydroxylase activity in the target organ may be necessary for the toxicity of a chemical to appear. As shown in studies by Nebert and colleagues [113], the magnitude of the basal and inducible levels of aryl hydrocarbon hydroxylase is influenced by genetic factors. Thus, treatment with 3-methylcholanthrene induces ovarian aryl hydrocarbon hydroxylase activity severalfold in mice response to enzyme induction by polycyclic hydrocarbons but not at all in a "nonresponsive" mouse strain. Under these conditions almost complete destruction of primordial oocytes has only been observed in the responsive mice [59,114]. Further, the detection of aryl hydrocarbon hydroxylase activity in bone marrow [115] has led to the suggestion that this may be the site at which toxic metabolites of benzene are formed [116]. Similarly, tissues such as mammary gland and pancreas, common sites for cancer, are both capable of activating benzo[a]pyrene.

Recent data have shown that the ultimate carcinogen of benzo[a]pyrene (BP) may be its diol-epoxide, 7,8-dihydro-7,8-dihydroxy-BP-9,10-oxide [117-119]. The toxic, mutagenic, and carcinogenic effects of benzo[a]pyrene are dependent on its metabolism by monooxygenases and related enzymes. The compound is enzymatically converted to epoxides, to at least four phenols and three quinones, to dihydrodiols, and to glutathione [120], glucuronide [121-123], and sulfate [104,123] conjugates. As mentioned earlier, there exist qualitative differences between the drug-metabolizing ability of the liver and other organs. These differences may also manifest themselves in directing the metabolic fate of potentially harmful compounds toward metabolic routes leading to tissue damage or protecting from it. Further experiments are obviously needed in order to obtain a satisfactory assessment of the full role of extrahepatic drug metabolism in relation to tissue damage.

In addition to the in situ formation of active intermediates, reactive metabolites may be transferred from the organ of formation to another organ, e.g., from the liver to remote target organs. The water-soluble conjugates of benzo[a]pyrene have been generally viewed as detoxication products; these products, primarily formed in the liver, are transported systemically to remote organs and are excreted in urine or feces. Recent studies indicate that benzo[a]pyrene glucuronides may not solely be detoxication products [124]. Instead, they may be converted to carcinogens by β-glucuronidase in extrahepatic tissues distant from their sites of formation [124].

B. β-Naphthylamine

The carcinogenicity of various arylamines and arylamides towards the liver
and urinary bladder has stimulated studies on the formation of reactive intermediates at the site of tumor formation. The N-oxidation of arylamines
and arylamides, catalyzed by monooxygenases in the endoplasmic reticulum
of liver and extrahepatic organs, has been regarded as an initial step for
hepatocarcinogenesis [cf. 125]. N-Hydroxy metabolites are subsequently
conjugated with, e.g., glucuronic acid and then excreted into urine. These
urinary glucuronides may be sufficiently electrophilic to react directly
with the epithelial cells of the bladder [126,127] or may be hydrolyzed to
N-hydroxy amines or N-hydroxy amides in the urinary tract; such compounds
can then be precursors for metabolic activation in the epithelial cells.
Another possibility is that reactive arylnitrenium ions, formed from the
N-hydroxy amines in acidic urine, may enter the epithelial cells and react
directly with critical cellular macromolecules, this reaction initiating carcinogenesis [128].

C. 4-Ipomeanol: A Lung-Toxic Furan Derivative

4-Ipomeanol [1-(3-furyl)-4-hydroxypentanone], a toxic furanoterpenoid
produced in mold-damaged sweet potatoes, reproducibly produces an acute,
specific pulmonary toxicity mediated by the pulmonary production of chemically reactive metabolites [129]. The highly reactive metabolite of this
naturally occurring furan derivative is primarily formed and covalently
bound in pulmonary nonciliated bronchiolar cells, and this process leads to
necrosis [130]. The toxic metabolite, possibly an epoxide, is formed in
situ, rather than reaching the lung by the general circulation. The lung
localization of drug-metabolizing enzyme activity is of prime interest since
it may help explain the often localized toxic effects of foreign compounds
within the lung, and it may help in developing a specific cytotoxin as a new
approach to chemotherapy for lung cancer.

V. RELATIONSHIP BETWEEN THE SITE OF FORMATION OF
     METABOLITE(S) AND THE LOCALIZATION OF TOXICITY

A. Formation of Active Metabolites in Extrahepatic Tissues
     and in situ Toxicity

In attempting to evaluate the significance of the biotransformation system
in organs with low metabolic activity, the intriguing question of the in situ
activation of chemicals has arisen. This type of activation might explain
the organ specificity of some carcinogens. Besides the activation of the
compound by a drug-metabolizing system, other types of activation mechanisms also exist which contribute to the toxic effects. The formation of

nitrosamines from amines and nitrite in the acidic pH of the stomach is one
example.

Nitrosamines are not carcinogenic by themselves but need to be
metabolically activated by the monooxygenase system to ultimate carcinogens. In initiating carcinogenic transformation in the cells, the concentration of the ultimate carcinogen (active intermediate) may play a
key role, since it determines the covalent binding to cellular macromolecules. However, not only the biotransformation of the compound
but also its overall disposition determines the final effect and target organs
of the chemical. Thus, evaluation of the tissue-specific carcinogenesis of
nitrosamines and nitrosamides showed a positive correlation between tumor
incidence due to presence of nitrosamines in various tissues and the metabolic activation, whereas the carcinogenesis of N-nitrosamides was determined primarily by the distribution of the compounds [131]. The nonspecific
cytoplasmic esterases may also regulate the carcinogenic effects of chemicals, depending on the administration route. One example is N-(acetoxy)-
methyl-N-methylnitrosamine, which is carcinogenic either to the stomach
or to the colon depending on whether it is administered intragastrically
or intraperitoneally: after intragastric administration the nonspecific esterases of the stomach release the alkylating agent. In contrast, N,N-
dimethylnitrosamine is mainly carcinogenic in the liver since it requires
metabolic activation by monooxygenases to produce the ultimate carcinogen.

B. Distribution of Active Products to Target Organs

The possibility exists that a compound can be metabolically activated in the
liver and the active intermediate transported to the target tissues. Generally the active intermediates have a very short half-life, and their transpor-
tation to other tissues in an active form is therefore questionable. However,
reactive metabolites of the brain carcinogen 3,3-dimethyl-1-phenyltriazene
are known to be transported from the activating tissue to the ultimate target
organ [131]. This compound can be metabolically activated in the liver by
oxidative N-demethylation to yield 3-methyl-1-phenyltriazene, which is a
directly acting alkylating agent unstable in aqueous media.

Many factors are known to influence the toxic reactions caused by
chemicals in extrahepatic tissues. The following list is a summary of these
factors:

1. Route of administration
2. Tissue distribution
3. Pharmacokinetic properties of the drug
4. Hepatic biotransformation—(a) Phase I versus Phase II reactions;
    (b) hepatic enzyme induction or inhibition
5. Biotransformation activity in the target organ

6. Stability of reactive intermediates; their transport from activating tissue to target organs
7. Secondary in situ activation in the target organ; hydrolysis of glucuronides
8. Repair mechanisms in the target organ

Even when extrahepatic toxicity is being judged, hepatic biotransformation activity may play a key role. For example, conjugation mechanisms in the liver may be enhanced to detoxify reactive intermediates. It is known that inhibition of the hepatic monooxygenase system increases the incidence of N-nitrosamine-induced extrahepatic tumors while the hepatic incidence is decreased [131]. The final factor, and one of the most important, regulating the expression of carcinogenic transformation is the role of DNA-repair mechanisms in the target cells [132].

VI. SIGNIFICANCE OF EXTRAHEPATIC DRUG METABOLISM

In this chapter we have evaluated the significance of extrahepatic drug metabolism to the organism both quantitatively and qualitatively. It is well established that extrahepatic tissues are capable of biotransformation, although the biological significance of these reactions is poorly understood. In global terms it is probable that extrahepatic metabolism has only a minor role in drug disposition. However, we have shown in this chapter that extrahepatic biotransformation can be greatly induced or activated [133,134] and that the degree of induction or activation also affects the elimination of the drugs in question. This phenomenon is well demonstrated by the studies of Conney and coworkers [84], who emphasized the significance of intestinal biotransformation. Therapeutic drugs are often administered orally, and thus the gastrointestinal tract is the first organ to come in contact with the chemical. Not only the intestinal wall but also the intestinal microflora may transform the compound enzymically, while the gastric fluids may act additionally in a nonenzymic manner. Thus, a drug may be at least partly converted to a metabolic product before even entering the portal veins. Further, as demonstrated by Josting and collaborators [135], the intestinal wall is actually capable of conjugating a major portion of the chemical administered. It is possible therefore that some compounds are inactivated to conjugated derivatives and excreted through the mucosal wall back to the intestinal lumen to be excreted out of the body.

Of much greater interest than purely pharmacological implications are other consequences of extrahepatic drug metabolism. The gastrointestinal tract, skin, and lungs form the portals of entry of drugs, pollutants, occupational chemicals, etc., into the body. Originally, drug-metabolizing enzymes were thought to have merely a defensive role since it was assumed that they only detoxified chemicals. Unfortunately, due to the multiplicity of the chemical structure of compounds entering the body, biotransformation reactions may also produce reactive intermediates. The kidneys have a role in the regulation of drug metabolism by excreting such compounds from the body. Although most compounds are in a water-soluble form before entering the kidneys, the kidneys are also capable of metabolizing xenobiotics. An inactive metabolite may be hydrolyzed by β-glucuronidase in the walls of the urinary tract, leading to the appearance of reactive metabolites in the urine.

Environmental xenobiotics enter the body in small quantities, but they still may be able to initiate toxic reactions due to metabolic activation. Since a threshold limit for carcinogenic/mutagenic transformation may not exist, it is possible that even low metabolic activity may yield reactive intermediates. The induction in extrahepatic tissues in some instances promotes the formation of mutagenic active intermediates. Lately some interesting studies have been conducted by Benditt [136] and by Juchau et al. [58], who have found that the aorta of rabbits, monkeys, and humans possesses aryl hydrocarbon hydroxylase activity. From these data they have hypothesized that environmental agents might also be converted to a reactive form in the aortic walls and consequently cause mutations in the smooth muscle cells and initiate the formation of a monoclonal atherosclerotic plaque. This model would even explain atherosclerosis as a disease caused by environmental pollution. Those endocrine organs participating in steroid biosynthesis, i.e., adrenal glands, testes, and ovaries, have relatively high cytochrome P-450 levels both in microsomal and mitochondrial fractions. The striking regional variation for human ovarian cancer, with a high incidence in industrialized countries, as well as an increase in incidence in recent years [137], underscores the possible importance of the metabolic activation of xenobiotics in the ovaries.

In future research the role of extrahepatic drug metabolism will, we hope, be more definitely established. Data for many organs are almost totally lacking, and the significance of biotransformation in some extrahepatic tissues remains to be clarified in terms of both drug disposition and initiation of tissue damage.

REFERENCES

1. E. Boyland, Proc. Roy. Soc. Med. 60:93 (1967).
2. R. Doll, Prevention of Cancer: Pointers for Epidemiology (The Rock Carling Fellowship 1967—Nuffield Provincial Hospitals Trust 1967). Whitefriars Press, London, 1967.
3. J. Higginson, Proc. 8th Can. Cancer Conf. p. 40 (1969).
4. K. W. Bock and D. Winne, Biochem. Pharmacol. 24:859 (1975).
5. J. R. Bend and G. E. R. Hook, in Reactions to Environmental Agents (Handbook of Physiology). American Physiological Soc., Bethesda, Md., 1977, p. 419.

6. B. B. Brodie, J. R. Gillette, and B. N. La Du, Ann. Rev. Biochem. 27:427 (1958).
7. R. W. Estabrook, J. R. Gillette, and K. C. Leibman (eds.), Microsomes and Drug Oxidations. Williams & Wilkins, Baltimore, 1973.
8. J. R. Fouts, in Methods in Pharmacology (A. Schwartz, ed.), Vol. 1. Appleton-Century-Crofts, New York, 1971, p. 287.
9. J. R. Gillette, Progr. Drug Res. 6:13 (1963).
10. J. R. Gillette, A. H. Conney, G. J. Cosmides, R. W. Estabrook, J. R. Fouts, and G. J. Mannering (eds.), Microsomes and Drug Oxidations. Academic Press, New York, 1969.
11. B. N. La Du, H. G. Mandel, and E. L. Way (eds.), Fundamentals of Drug Metabolism and Disposition. Williams & Wilkins, Baltimore, 1971.
12. D. V. Parke, The Biochemistry of Foreign Compounds. Pergamon Press, Elmsford, N.Y., 1968.
13. J. W. DePierre and G. Dallner, Biochim. Biophys. Acta 415:411 (1975).
14. J. W. DePierre and L. Ernster, Ann. Rev. Biochem. 46:201 (1976).
15. R. W. Estabrook, J. Werringloer, B. S. S. Masters, H. Jonen, T. Matsubara, R. Ebel, D. O'Keefe, and J. A. Peterson, in The Structural Basis of Membrane Function (Y. Hatefi and L. Djavadi-Ohaniance, eds.). Academic Press, New York, 1976, p. 429.
16. H. Vainio, On the topology and synthesis of drug-metabolizing enzymes in hepatic endoplasmic reticulum. Dissertation, University of Turku, Turku, Finland, 1973.
17. H. Vainio, in Proc. 6th Int. Congr. Pharmacol., Helsinki, 1975, p. 53.
18. A. Aitio, Extrahepatic microsomal drug metabolism. Dissertation, University of Turku, Turku, Finland, 1973.
19. A. Aitio and J. Marniemi, in Extrahepatic Drug Metabolism (T. E. Gram, ed.). Spectrum Publns., Holliswood, N.Y., 1980, in press.
20. G. J. Dutton, in Handbook of Experimental Pharmacology: Concepts in Biochemical Pharmacology, Part II (B. B. Brodie and J. R. Gillette, eds.). Springer, New York, 1971, Vol. 28, p. 378.
21. G. J. Dutton (ed.), Glucuronic Acid: Free and Combined—Chemistry, Biochemistry, Pharmacology and Medicine. Academic Press, New York, 1966.
22. S. A. Atlas, S. S. Thorgeirsson, A. R. Boobis, K. Kumaki, and D. W. Nebert, Biochem. Pharmacol. 24:2111 (1975).
23. M. K. Buening and M. R. Franklin, Drug Metab. Dispos. 4:556 (1976).
24. R. S. Chhabra, R. J. Pohl, and J. R. Fouts, Drug Metab. Dispos. 2:443 (1974).
25. D. L. Cinti and M. R. Montgomery, Life Sci. 18:1223 (1976).
26. J. W. Greiner, R. E. Kramer, D. A. Robinson, W. J. Canad, and H. D. Colby, Biochem. Pharmacol. 25:951 (1976).

27. E. Hietanen and H. Vainio, Arch. Environ. Contam. Toxicol. 4:201 (1976).
28. H. Hoensch, C. H. Woo, S. B. Ruffin, and R. Schmid, Gastro-enterology 70:1063 (1976).
29. G. E. R. Hook, J. K. Haseman, and G. W. Lucier, Chem.-Biol. Interactions 10:199 (1975).
30. S. V. Jakobsson and D. L. Cinti, J. Pharmacol. Exp. Ther. 185:226 (1973).
31. D. P. Jones, S. Orrenius, and S. V. Jakobsson, in Extrahepatic Drug Metabolism (T. E. Gram, ed.), Spectrum Publns., Holliswood, N.Y., 1980, in press.
32. W. Kuenzig, W. Tkaczevski, J. J. Kamm, A. H. Conney, and J. J. Burns, J. Pharmacol. Exp. Ther. 201:527 (1977).
33. R. H. Menard, S. A. Latif, and J. L. Purvis, Endocrinology 97:1587 (1975).
34. S. Orrenius, Å. Ellin, S. V. Jakobsson, H. Thor, D. L. Cinti, J. B. Schenkman, and R. W. Estabrook, Drug Metab. Dispos. 1:350 (1973).
35. R. J. Pohl, R. M. Philpot, and J. R. Fouts, Pharmacologist 16:322 (1974).
36. H. Remmer, Proc. 6th Int. Congr. Pharmacol. 6:67 (1975).
37. H. A. Sasame, M. M. Ames, and S. D. Nelson, Biochem. Biophys. Res. Commun. 78:919 (1977).
38. B. C. Shanley, V. A. Percy, and A. C. Neethling, SA Med. J. 51:458 (1977).
39. S. J. Stohs, R. C. Grafstrom, M. D. Burke, P. W. Moldeus, and S. Orrenius, Arch. Biochem. Biophys. 177:105 (1976).
40. S. J. Stohs, R. C. Grafstrom, M. D. Burke, and S. Orrenius, Drug Metab. Dispos. 4:517 (1976).
41. B. Testa and P. Jenner, Drug Metabolism: Chemical and Biochemical Aspects. Dekker, New York, 1976.
42. J. M. Tredger and R. S. Chhabra, Xenobiotica 7:481 (1977).
43. J. M. Tredger, R. S. Chhabra, and J. R. Fouts, Drug Metab. Dispos. 4:451 (1976).
44. H. Vainio, Xenobiotica 3:715 (1973).
45. R. H. Wickramasinghe, Enzyme 19:348 (1975).
46. E. Ackermann, K. Richter, and S. Sage, Biochem. Pharmacol. 25:1557 (1976).
47. C. L. Litterst, E. G. Mimnaugh, P. L. Reagan, and T. E. Gram, Drug Metab. Dispos. 3:259 (1975).
48. C. L. Litterst, E. G. Mimnaugh, R. L. Reagan, and T. E. Gram, Life Sci. 17:813 (1975).
49. C. L. Litterst, E. G. Mimnaugh, and T. E. Gram, Biochem. Pharmacol. 26:749 (1977).
50. O. Pelkonen, E. H. Kaltiala, T. K. I. Larmi, and N. T. Karki, Clin. Pharmacol. Ther. 14:840 (1973).

51. H. Vainio, J. Marniemi, M. Parkki, and R. Luoma, in Biological Reactive Intermediates (D. J. Jollow, J. J. Kocsis, R. Snyder, and H. Vainio, eds.). Plenum Press, New York, 1977, p. 251.

52. A. P. Alvares, D. R. Bickers, and A. Kappas, Proc. Nat. Acad. Sci. U.S. 70:1321 (1973).

53. A. P. Alvares and A. Kappas, Clin. Pharmacol. Ther. 22:809 (1977).

54. A. H. L. Chuang and E. Bresnick, Cancer Res. 36:4125 (1976).

55. J. A. Cohn, A. P. Alvares, and A. Kappas, J. Exp. Med. 145:1607 (1977).

56. K. Hartiala, Physiol. Rev. 53:496 (1973).

57. Z. M. Iqbal, M. E. Varnes, A. Yoshida, and S. S. Epstein, Cancer Res. 37:1011 (1977).

58. M. R. Juchau, J. A. Bond, and E. P. Benditt, Proc. Nat. Acad. Sci. U.S. 73:3723 (1976).

59. D. R. Mattison and S. S. Thorgeirsson, Biochem. Pharmacol. 26: 909 (1977).

60. M. R. Montgomery and D. L. Cinti, Mol. Pharmacol. 13:60 (1970).

61. D. W. Nebert and H. V. Gelboin, Arch. Biochem. Biophys. 134:76 (1969).

62. A. J. Paine and A. E. M. McLean, Biochem. Pharmacol. 22:2875 (1975).

63. J. B. Schenkman, K. M. Robie, and I. Jansson, in Biological Reactive Intermediates (D. J. Jollow, J. J. Kocsis, R. Snyder, and H. Vainio, eds.). Plenum Press, New York, 1977, p. 83.

64. S. J. Stohs, R. C. Grafstrom, M. D. Burke, and S. Orrenius, Arch. Biochem. Biophys. 179:71 (1977).

65. P. Uotila and J. Marniemi, Biochem. Pharmacol. 25:2323 (1976).

66. M. Watanabe, K. Konno, and H. Sato, Gann 66:123 (1973).

67. P. J. Wiebel, J. C. Leutz, and H. V. Gelboin, Arch. Biochem. Biophys. 154:292 (1973).

68. F. J. Wiebel, J. C. Leutz, and H. V. Gelboin, J. Invest. Dermatol. 64:184 (1975).

68a. A. Pannatier, P. Jenner, B. Testa, and J. C. Etter, Drug Metab. Rev. 8:319 (1978).

69. N. G. Zampaglione and G. J. Mannering, J. Pharmacol. Exp. Ther. 185:676 (1973).

70. A. Aitio, Anal. Biochem. 85:488 (1978).

71. V. Ullrich, Arzneim. Forsch. 27:1821 (1977).

72. M. O. James, G. L. Foureman, F. C. Law, and J. R. Bend, Drug Metab. Dispos. 5:19 (1976).

73. M. O. James, G. L. Foureman, F. C. Law, and J. R. Bend, Biochem. Pharmacol. 25:187 (1977).

74. F. Oesch, H. Glatt, and H. Schmassmann, Biochem. Pharmacol. 26: 603 (1977).

75. A. Aitio, H. Vainio, and O. Hänninen, FEBS Lett. 124:237 (1972).

76. O. Hänninen and A. Aitio, Biochem. Pharmacol. 17:2307 (1968).
77. E. I. Ciaccio and H. DeVera, Biochem. Pharmacol. 25:985 (1975).
78. H. Vadi, P. Moldéus, J. Capdevila, and S. Orrenius, Cancer Res. 35:2082 (1975).
79. A. Aitio, Int. J. Biochem. 5:325 (1974).
80. R. Grafström, S. J. Stohs, M. D. Burke, P. Moldéus, and S. Orrenius, Microsomes and Drug Oxidation (V. Ullrich, I. Roots, A. Hildebrandt, R. W. Estabrook, and A. H. Conney, eds.). Pergamon Press, Oxford, 1977, p. 667.
81. T. C. Campbell and J. R. Hayes, Pharmacol. Rev. 26:171 (1971).
82. E. Agradi, C. Spagnuolo, and C. Galli, Pharmacol. Res. Commun. 7:469 (1975).
83. A. H. Conney, E. S. Pantuck, K.-C. Hsiao, R. Kuntzman, A. P. Alvares, and A. Kappas, Fed. Proc. 36:1647 (1977).
84. A. H. Conney, E. J. Pantuck, R. Kuntzman, A. Kappas, K. E. Anderson, and A. P. Alvares, Clin. Pharmacol. Ther. 22:707 (1977).
85. E. Hietanen and M. Laitinen, Biochem. Pharmacol. 27:1095 (1978).
86. R. Kuntzman, E. J. Pantuck, S. A. Kaplan, and A. H. Conney, Clin. Pharmacol. Ther. 22:757 (1977).
87. W. D. Loub, L. W. Wattenberg, and D. W. Davis, J. Nat. Cancer Inst. 54:985 (1975).
88. E. J. Pantuck, K.-C. Hsiao, A. H. Conney, W. A. Earland, A. Kappas, K. E. Anderson, and A. P. Alvares, Science 194:1055 (1974).
89. E. J. Pantuck, K.-C. Hsiao, R. Kuntzman, and A. H. Conney, Science 187:744 (1975).
90. E. J. Pantuck, R. Kuntzman, and A. H. Conney, in New Concepts in Safety Evaluation (M. A. Meheman, R. E. Shapiro, and H. Blumenthal, eds.). Halstedt Press, Washington, D.C., 1976, p. 345.
91. P. Uotila, Res. Commun. Chem. Pathol. Pharmacol. 17:101 (1977).
92. H. L. Falk, in Reactions to Environmental Agents (Handbook of Physiology). American Physiological Soc., Bethesda, Md., 1977, p. 199.
93. R. M. Welch, J. Cavallito, and A. Loh, Toxicol. Appl. Pharmacol. 23:749 (1972).
94. R. M. Welch, A. Loh, and A. H. Conney, Life Sci. 10:215 (1971).
95. F. J. Akin and J. F. Benner, Toxicol. Appl. Pharmacol. 35:331 (1976).
96. R. K. Abrahamson and J. J. Hutton, Cancer Res. 35:23 (1975).
97. P. G. Holt and D. Keast, Experientia 29:1004 (1972).
98. J. Van Cantfort and J. Gielen, Biochem. Pharmacol. 24:1253 (1975).
99. E. T. Cantrell, G. A. Warr, D. L. Busbee, and R. R. Martin, J. Clin. Invest. 52:1881 (1973).
100. O. Pelkonen, P. Jouppila, and N. T. Kärki, Toxicol. Appl. Pharmacol. 23:399 (1972).
101. R. M. Welch, Y. E. Harrison, B. W. Commi, P. J. Poppers, M. Finster, and A. H. Conney, Clin. Pharmacol. Ther. 10:100 (1969).
102. G. M. Cohen, P. Uotila, J. Hartiala, E.-M. Suolinna, N. Simberg, and O. Pelkonen, Cancer Res. 37:2147 (1977).

103. H. Vainio, P. Uotila, J. Hartiala, and O. Pelkonen, Res. Commun. Chem. Pathol. Pharmacol. 13:259 (1976).

104. G. M. Cohen, S. M. Haws, B. P. Moore, and J. W. Bridges, Biochem. Pharmacol. 25:2561 (1976).

105. K. Pal, P. L. Grover, and P. Sims, Biochem. Soc. Trans. 3:1974 (1975).

106. P. L. Grover, A. Hewer, K. Pal, and P. Sims, Int. J. Cancer 18:1 (1976).

107. C. C. Harris, V. M. Genta, A. L. Frank, D. G. Kaufman, L. A. Barrett, E. M. McDowell, and B. F. Trump, Nature 252:68 (1974).

108. S. N. Hunt, W. J. Jusko, and A. M. Yurchak, Clin. Pharmacol. Ther. 19:546 (1976).

109. J. M. Perel, M. Shostak, E. Gann, S. J. Kantor, and A. H. Glassman, in Pharmacokinetics of Psychoactive Drugs: Drug Levels and Clinical Response (L. A. Gottschalk and E. Merlis, eds.). Spectrum Publns., Holliswood, N.Y., 1976, p. 229.

110. R. E. Vestal, A. H. Norris, J. D. Tobin, B. H. Cohen, N. W. Shock, and A. Andres, Clin. Pharmacol. Ther. 18:425 (1975).

111. R. P. Batzinger, E. Bueding, B. S. Reddy, and J. H. Weisburger, Cancer Res. 38:608 (1978).

112. R. R. Scheline, Excerpta Medica Int. Congr. Ser. 254:35 (1971).

113. D. W. Nebert, R. C. Levitt, N. M. Jensen, G. H. Lambert, and J. S. Felton, Arch. Toxicol. 39:109 (1977).

114. D. R. Mattison and S. S. Thorgeisson, Lancet i:187 (1978).

115. L. S. Andrews, B. R. Sonawane, and S. J. Yaffe, Res. Commun. Chem. Pathol. Pharmacol. 15:319 (1976).

116. R. Snyder, E. W. Lee, J. J. Kocsis, and C. M. Witmer, Life Sci. 21:1709 (1977).

117. J. Kapitulnik, P. G. Wislocki, W. Levin, H. Yagi, D. M. Jerina, and A. H. Conney, Cancer Res. 38:354 (1978).

118. M. Koreeda, P. D. Moore, P. G. Wislocki, W. Levin, and A. H. Conney, Science 199:778 (1978).

119. P. Sims, P. L. Grover, A. Swaisland, K. Pal, and A. Hewer, Nature 252:326 (1974).

120. N. Nemoto and H. V. Gelboin, Arch. Biochem. Biophys. 170:739 (1975).

121. N. Nemoto and H. V. Gelboin, Biochem. Pharmacol. 25:1221 (1976).

122. N. Nemoto and S. Takayama, Cancer Res. 37:4125 (1977).

123. N. Nemoto, S. Takayama, and H. V. Gelboin, Biochem. Pharmacol. 26:1825 (1977).

124. N. Kinoshita and H. V. Gelboin, Science 199:307 (1978).

125. J. H. Weisburger and E. K. Weisburger, Pharmacol. Rev. 25:1 (1973).

126. C. C. Irving, in Metabolic Conjugation and Metabolic Hydrolysis (W. H. Fishman, ed.), Vol. 1. Academic Press, New York, 1970, p. 53.

127. C. C. Irving, D. H. Janss, and L. T. Russell, Cancer Res. 31:387 (1971).

128. F. F. Kadlubar, J. A. Miller, and E. C. Miller, Cancer Res. 37: 805 (1977).

129. M. R. Boyd, Environ. Health Perspect. 16:127 (1976).

130. M. R. Boyd, Nature 269:713 (1977).

131. H. Bartsch, G. P. Margison, C. Malaveille, A. M. Camus, G. Brun, J. M. Margison, G. F. Kolar, and M. Weissler, Arch. Toxicol. 39: 51 (1977).

132. J. L. Van Lancker, in Current Topics in Pathology (E. Grundmann and W. H. Kirsten, eds.). Springer, New York, 1977, p. 65.

133. L. W. Wattenberg, Gastroenterology 51:932 (1966).

134. L. W. Wattenberg, J. L. Leong, and P. J. Strand, Cancer Res. 22: 1120 (1962).

135. D. Josting, D. Winne, and K. W. Bock, Biochem. Pharmacol. 25: 613 (1976).

136. E. A. Benditt, Sci. Amer. p. 74 (Feb. 1977).

137. J. Waterhouse, P. Correa, C. Muir, and J. Powell, Cancer Incidence in Five Continents. IARC Scientific Publns. No. 15, Lyons, France, 1976, p. 1.

Chapter 6

DEVELOPMENTAL DRUG METABOLISM

Olavi Pelkonen

Department of Pharmacology
University of Oulu
Oulu, Finland

The developmental patterns of drug metabolism in common laboratory animals can be broadly divided into two general classes, namely, those pathways which develop rapidly after birth and those which develop only slowly. Although oxidative pathways are in general poorly developed prenatally, some conjugation reactions are well established in the fetus during the first half of pregnancy. The principal difference between humans and common laboratory animals is that the human fetus can oxidize foreign compounds to a considerable extent. This ability resides mainly in the liver and in the adrenal glands which possess cytochrome P-450-linked electron transport chains.

The hepatic and adrenal oxidative enzyme systems of the human fetus seem to be constitutive by nature, whereas the placental system is almost exclusively present in the placentas of smoking mothers. There are great differences between hepatic, adrenal, and placental enzyme systems with respect to substrate selectivity and activity, spectral interactions, and apparent inducibility by exogenous substances.

Recent studies indicate that the ontogenetic development of the monooxygenase systems seems to be more complicated than expected, with various enzymes emerging (and some disappearing) in a definite pattern. The temporal changes of different forms of enzymes and even their inducibilities may be regulated quite independently from each other and give rise to definitive patterns for each animal species.

Possible consequences of this fetal drug-metabolizing capacity are changes in steady-state levels of substances, accumulation of polar metabolites, steroid-xenobiotic interactions, and the formation of toxic intermediates that might lead, for example, to teratogenesis and transplacental carcinogenesis.

I. INTRODUCTION

Drugs and other compounds foreign to the body are metabolized by enzyme
systems in the liver and other tissues. In the adult metabolism is the most
important way by which the body gets rid of exogenous (and in many cases,
also endogenous) lipophilic substances. However, as is evident, this activity may change as a function of age, and the first studies that sought to
elucidate the development of xenobiotic-metabolizing enzymes were published almost 30 years ago. Since then, the majority of studies have indicated that the fetus as well as the newborn is poorly equipped with xenobiotic-
metabolizing enzymes, with obvious implications for the pharmacokinetics
of foreign compounds in the body. On the other hand, other studies have
revealed that senescent organisms may be less able to metabolize foreign
compounds than are adults in their prime. These early studies led to the
revival, with respect to drug metabolism, of E. H. Haeckel's principle
(1866) that the ontogenetic development of an individual repeats the phylo-
genetic development of the species. This "recapitulation" hypothesis was
further supported by evidence showing that fish and amphibians were relatively poor in metabolizing foreign substances [1]. However, recent studies
indicate that this picture might be too simple, and considerable interest is
currently centered on the ontogenetic regulation of drug-metabolizing enzymes in animals and humans.

Because developmental aspects of the drug-metabolizing enzyme systems in nonprimate mammals have been studied for more than 20 years and a large number of reviews on various aspects of this subject are available [2-20], I will concentrate in this chapter mainly on general patterns, on regulatory aspects, and on possible implications of fetal and neonatal drug metabolism. I will also refer mostly to reviews rather than original articles.

II. PATTERNS AND PATHWAYS OF FETAL AND NEONATAL DRUG METABOLISM

A. Oxidative Enzymes

It is best to start this presentation with a schematic diagram (Fig. 1) which shows ontogenetic development of drug-metabolizing enzymes in various species and with various substrates. The curves shown are based, at least in part, on experimental evidence, and although some imagination has been used in constructing them, they illustrate typical findings in developmental drug metabolism.

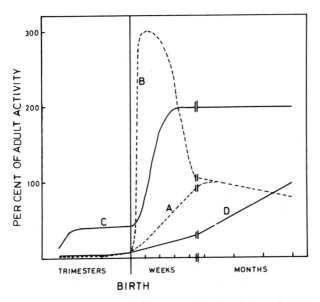

FIGURE 1   Patterns of ontogenetic development of drug metabolism for human (solid lines) and for nonprimate mammalian species (dashed lines). For explanation, see text.

1. Animal fetuses and neonates

Curve A in Fig. 1 summarizes the development of several drug-oxidizing and -reducing activities in the rat and other nonprimate species. After the pioneering reports of Jondorf et al. [21] and Fouts and Adamson [22], it has become increasingly clear that many laboratory animal species, including the rat, guinea pig, mouse, rabbit, hamster, and ferret are deficient in hepatic microsomal drug-oxidizing activity associated with the cytochrome P-450-linked microsomal electron transport chain during the early stages of their development [18-20; cf. references therein]. With a few exceptions, these species have a very low capacity to oxidize drugs and other foreign compounds until after birth. Adult levels of xenobiotic metabolism are not observed until the animal is at least several weeks old. Although curve A is applicable to most drug-oxidizing and -reducing pathways in nonprimate species, there is a small number of pathways or reactions in any species differing from this general development curve, especially in the postnatal development of drug metabolism. Curve B represents these few pathways. The maturation is rapid, occurring within a few days after birth [e.g., see Ref. 23].

Although results obtained in different laboratories vary somewhat from each other with respect to the absolute activities of drug-oxidizing enzymes during different phases of development and with respect to the pattern of development, it may be concluded that the fetuses of common laboratory species are deficient in both the cytochrome P-450-linked electron transport chain and related enzyme activities. However, the deficiency is never absolute since the measurable activity of drug-oxidizing enzymes in the fetus represents only a few percent, at most, of the adult levels.

2. Human fetus and neonate

During recent years it has become increasingly clear that the human fetus is able to metabolize foreign compounds, unlike fetuses of common laboratory species [7, 8, 11, 20].

Curve C in Fig. 1 represents the development of a number of drug-oxidizing enzyme activities and cytochrome P-450 enzyme in human fetal and newborn liver. Naturally, the postnatal part of the curve is inferred from pharmacokinetic studies. This curve seems to be completely different from curve A, which is typical for nonprimate species. On the other hand, when the different time scales for the postnatal development of humans and small laboratory animals are taken into account, one can speculate that the postnatal portions of curves B and C are not too dissimilar.

The fourth type of curve (D) in Fig. 1 represents the development of cytochrome P-448- or P-450-linked enzyme activities in humans. This curve somewhat resembles curve A, typical for the rat and other species. Again, the postnatal development of the enzyme activity is inferred from the pharmacokinetic studies of a few drugs. It thus appears that there are certain similarities in postnatal maturation of drug metablism between human beings and laboratory animal species as far as patterns are concerned.

An important question is whether or not the species differences (especially in prenatal drug metabolism) observed between the human fetus and the fetuses of common laboratory animals are real or only apparent, being a consequence of differences in the gestation period, in the development stages of gestation, or in the maturity of fetuses of various species. When one compares the period of embryogenesis and the approximate time of appearance of drug-oxidizing enzyme systems in the fetal liver in different species, one can clearly see that drug metabolism appears in the human fetus in late embryogenesis but some time after that period in various laboratory animal species. This would indicate that there is indeed a real species difference [20]. Since the human fetus and neonate seem to differ considerably from animal fetuses and neonates, it is worthwhile to give a general outline of drug-metabolizing enzyme systems in human fetal tissues and placenta. A more detailed description can be found in the author's earlier review [20], where many original references are also to be found.

3. Tissue distribution

Typical components of a drug-oxidizing monooxygenase system, namely, cytochrome P-450 and NADPH-cytochrome c (P-450) reductase, have been detected in the liver, adrenal glands, and placenta (Table 1) [20; see references therein]. The activity of NADPH-cytochrome c reductase is of the same order of magnitude in the three tissues studied, but there are large differences in the amount of cytochrome P-450 present. Slight drug-metabolizing activity has also been detected in kidneys, lungs, and intestine, but this activity is sufficiently low to prevent the reliable detection and characterization of cytochrome P-450 [20].

Studies on carbon monoxide (CO)- and ethyl isocyanide (EIS)-induced spectra of cytochrome P-450 in fetal liver, adrenal glands, and placenta have shown the hemoprotein to have characteristic peaks in the same wavelength region as found in experimental animals and man, about 450 nm (CO) and 430 and 445 nm (EIS). The most notable difference between the tissues was the finding that with adrenal microsomes the peak of the CO-induced difference spectrum is located at 446-448 nm whereas with hepatic and placental microsomes the peak was located at about 450 nm or even higher.

4. Substrate selectivity

The monooxygenase systems in various tissues differ from each other with respect to substrate selectivity, relative activity towards different substrates, drug-induced spectral interactions, and inducibility by exogenous substances (Table 1). The hepatic monooxygenase system catalyzes the oxidative metabolism of a wide variety of compounds, including drugs such as aminopyrine, ethylmorphine, hexobarbital, diazepam, chlorpromazine,

TABLE 1
Some Characteristics of Drug-Oxidizing Monooxygenase Systems
in Human Fetal Liver, Adrenal Glands, and Placenta

Parameter	Fetal liver	Adrenal glands	Placenta	Adult liver
Cytochrome P-450[a]	3–11 (0.3)	12–38 (1.7)	? (<0.1)	10–20 (0.6)
Oxidation of xenobiotics				
Aminopyrine	++	+	0	++++
Aniline	+++	+	0	++++
7-Ethoxycoumarin	++	+	+ to ++++	++++
Benzo[a]pyrene	+	++	0 to ++++	++++
Oxidation of steroids	Numerous substrates	Numerous substrates	Fewer substrates	Numerous substrates
Oxidation of fatty acids	yes	not studied	no	yes
Spectral interactions with:				
Hexobarbital	I or RI	no	no	I
Tetrachloroethane	I	no	no	I
Aniline	II	II	II	II
Dehydroepiandrosterone	I	II	I	I
Inducibility by:				
Phenobarbital	possible	no	(in smokers?)	yes
Polycyclic hydrocarbons	no	no	yes	yes

[a] nmol cytochrome P-450/g wet tissue. Numbers in parentheses indicate nmol cytochrome P-450/mg microsomal protein.

and desmethylimipramine, dye intermediates such as N-methylaniline and aniline, carcinogens such as benzo[a]pyrene, and pesticides such as aldrin, and also the reduction of para-nitrobenzoic acid and Neoprontosil. The adrenal monooxygenase system also catalyzes the oxidative and reductive metabolism of several substrates, although somewhat more uncertain results have been obtained and fewer compounds have been studied. The placental metabolism of foreign compounds has been extensively studied; but as far as microsomal drug metabolism is concerned, only a few oxidative pathways have been detected, and these almost exclusively in placentas from smoking mothers. More recent studies indicate that some compounds, for example, 7-ethoxycoumarin, can be metabolized by placentas from nonsmokers, thus suggesting the presence of two drug-oxidizing enzyme systems in the placenta—a "constitutive" system and a cigarette-smoke-inducible system [24,25].

5. Spectral interactions

The addition to liver microsomes of various substances, such as hexobarbital, aniline, or n-butanol, causes different types of spectral changes which have been termed type I, type II, and reverse type I (RI), respectively [26]. The microsomes from liver, adrenal glands, and placenta all interact with different xenobiotics, steroids, and other compounds, but there are major differences in the type and magnitude of the spectral interactions observed for the various tissues. Especially interesting are differences between the three tissues in the production of type I spectral changes. Drugs and other xenobiotics which give a type I spectral change with rat liver microsomes interact with microsomes from fetal liver but not with those from adrenal glands or placenta. Notable differences among liver, adrenal glands, and placenta are also detected with respect to steroid-induced type I interactions (Table 1). These differences in spectral interactions imply that significant differences exist among the three tissues in the catalytic activity of cytochrome P-450, and this is indeed the case when one compares spectral interactions to substrate selectivity and to steroid metabolism data (Table 1) [20].

On the basis of substrate selectivity and spectral interaction studies with fetal liver, adrenal glands, and placenta, it is possible to formulate the following overall picture. The liver is the most capable and also the least specific tissue for metabolizing xenobiotics; the adrenal glands probably are more restrictive in their substrate selectivity, although not necessarily in activity towards some substrates; and the placenta has only a few drug-oxidizing pathways, at least some of which are detectable almost exclusively in the placenta of smoking mothers. As a result it is probable that most xenobiotics are not metabolized in the placenta but are subject to oxidative and reductive metabolism in the fetal liver and adrenal glands.

6. Comparison with adult monooxygenase systems

Generally, fetal hepatic levels of monooxygenase components and related enzyme activities vary in the second trimester of gestation from 20 to 50% of adult hepatic levels [27], although even higher percentages have been observed [28,29]. The liver, however, represents some 4-5% of the fetal weight but only about 2% of the adult weight. As a consequence, the activities of these enzymes in the fetus may approach those of human adults on a body weight basis. With respect to some substrates, the fetal adrenal gland appears to be even more active than the fetal liver [30,31]. Also, fetal adrenal glands are relatively larger than the corresponding adult organ, and it must be concluded that they may contribute significantly to drug oxidation in the human fetus. Many studies have indicated that the characteristics of fetal enzymes closely resembled those of enzymes in adult human and laboratory animal liver with respect to cofactor requirements, microsomal location, substrate interactions, and inhibition [32,33]. However, other evidence has indicated that the fetal hepatic P-450 system differs qualitatively from that found in adult liver. First, the capacity of the human fetal liver to metabolize benzo[a]pyrene was only some 2-4% of the adult capacity, whereas the percentages for many other substrates ranged from 20 to 40% or even higher [27-29]. Second, a developmental change in the apparent kinetic properties of drug-oxidizing enzymes in the human liver was found, indicating qualitative differences between fetal and adult enzymes [34]. Third, some drug-induced spectral interactions differ between fetus and adult [35,36]. This evidence can all be taken to indicate qualitative differences between fetal and adult hepatic cytochrome P-450 systems, but how these differences are reflected in the catalytic properties of the enzyme is not entirely clear. It is apparent, nevertheless, that the fetal hepatic P-450 system seems to resemble that from the livers of control or phenobarbital-treated rats rather than from animals receiving polycyclic hydrocarbons and, consequently, its catalytic spectrum can be expected to be wide.

7. Human newborn infants

Table 2 contains data on the in vivo metabolism of selected substances by human newborn infants, children, and adults [15,18-18b]. The most notable finding, as pointed out by Neims et al. [18], is that the ability of the newborn to metabolize phenytoin or phenobarbital is only slightly less than the adult capacity. In contrast there is a marked difference in the disposition of caffeine and theophylline with age. Caffeine is metabolized by the cytochrome P-448 or P_1-450-linked enzyme system, as shown by the inducibility of caffeine metabolism by 3-methylcholanthrene [37]. These findings are in agreement with earlier studies which showed the human fetus to be deficient in metabolizing activity toward benzo[a]pyrene, a typical substrate for 3-methylcholanthrene-inducible monooxygenases [27,31]. With respect to reaction pathways, no metabolic route listed in Table 2 (except perhaps

TABLE 2
Selected Substances Metabolized in vivo by the Human Newborn, Children, and Adults

Substance	Reaction pathways suggested by in vivo metabolites	Half-life (hr) in:				
		Premature neonates	Full-term neonates		Children (1 yr)	Adults
			1st week	2nd week		
Phenytoin	Aromatic hydroxylation, epoxidation, epoxide hydration, glucuronidation	75	21	8	6	11-31
Phenobarbital	Aromatic hydroxylation, epoxidation, epoxide hydration, side chain oxidation, glucuronidation	--	200	100	50	100
Theophylline	N-demethylation	30	--	--	3.4	6.7
Caffeine	N-demethylation	36-144	← 32-149 →			4-5

Source: Data from Refs. 15, 18, 18a, and 18b.

glucuronidation) is at variance with the drug metabolism studies performed in vitro in human fetal tissue preparations or in human neonatal tissue preparations [38]. A good in vitro/in vivo correlation would therefore appear to exist.

B. Conjugation Reactions

Early studies [39-41] suggested that glucuronidation, like drug oxidation, was deficient during fetal and neonatal periods. Later studies, however, have shown that the development of glucuronidation is dependent upon species, strain, and substrate studied [42; cf. references therein]. For example, Burchell [43] found that in ASH/TO-strain mice, UDP-glucuronyltransferase activity towards ortho-aminophenol in 14-day fetal liver was at the adult level, whereas the activity of the same samples toward estriol was less than 1% of adult activity.

Glucuronic acid conjugation is the most thoroughly studied pathway, but some investigations have been carried out on the ontogenetic development of other conjugation reactions. For example, bilirubin UDP-glucosyltransferase activity [44], glycine conjugation [45], the conjugation of glutathione with sulfobromophthalein [46], and sulfotransferase activity [47] all are low or undetectable in liver and some other tissues of fetal or neonatal rodents. Thus most conjugation pathways are poorly developed in the fetuses of any one species, but this is found less consistently in such pathways than in drug oxidation reactions. Some species or strains are well equipped for glucuronic acid conjugation at the time of birth and even before.

Most studies on glucuronic acid conjugation by human fetal tissues demonstrate very low or absent activities using para-nitrophenol, ortho-aminophenol, 1-naphthol, and 4-methylumbelliferone as substrates [20; cf. references therein]. On the other hand, conjugation reactions such as conjugations with glutathione [48] or glycine [45] are fairly well developed in fetal tissues. The coupled development of hydroxylation and glucuronide conjugation [49] has been suggested by some studies but denied by others [42]. The latter studies show that the cytochrome P-450-linked enzyme system may develop before the UDP-glucuronyltransferase system does in human fetal liver and that these two systems are not necessarily coupled during human ontogenetic development. The presence of large amounts of sulfate and glucuronide conjugates of steroids in human fetal tissues and excreta (bile, amniotic fluid) points to active conjugative enzymes, but whether or not these steroid-conjugating enzymes also attack xenobiotics is not known [50].

C. Ultrastructural Studies

In an adult liver, drug-oxidizing enzymes are associated with the presence of smooth endoplasmic reticulum (SER) [51]. However, it has been reported that the fetal hepatocyte from rabbits [52,53], mice [54], and rats [55] contains little SER in comparison with the adult and that the SER appears only after birth. These results on liver ultrastructure therefore support the belief that in laboratory animals the major increase in drug-oxidizing activity occurs after birth.

Zamboni [56] studied the developmental histology of human fetal liver and found that the SER appears in hepatocytes around the third month of gestation with concomitant deposits of glycogen and iron. Interestingly, the time of appearance of the SER coincided with the appearance of drug-oxidizing enzymes in the human fetal liver [57]. Later studies showed that the appearance of SER in human fetal liver occurs much earlier than in animal fetal livers [58], in agreement with drug metabolism data.

D. Animal Models for Human Fetal Drug Metabolism

The lack of a suitable animal model for human fetal drug metabolism is at present one of the most serious hindrances in fetal pharmacology. In this respect nonhuman primates seem to resemble humans closely. For example, recent studies on the stumptail monkey and rhesus monkey revealed a considerable drug oxidation capacity in early gestation [30,59,60]. In agreement with these findings, Quattropani et al. [61] detected the presence of SER in fetal stumptail monkey liver. It is thus possible for nonhuman primates to be used as models in studying fetal drug metabolism and pharmacokinetics, although the high costs involved make large-scale studies impracticable.

III. ARYL HYDROCARBON HYDROXYLASE ACTIVITY IN FETAL TISSUES AND PLACENTA

Aryl hydrocarbon hydroxylase (AHH) must be dealt with separately from other drug-oxidizing activities because, besides its importance in carcinogenesis, mutagenesis, teratogenesis, and tissue lesions, it is an extremely useful probe in studying the characteristics of drug-metabolizing monooxygenase systems.

Practically all in vitro studies point to a general lack of this enzyme system in the tissues of fetal animals and to a gradual rise to adult levels after birth [20,62; cf. references therein]; also, the inducibility of AHH in fetal tissues changes as a function of fetal age. In any case, basal levels of AHH in fetal tissues are always extremely low (or not detectable) and even after induction do not usually reach adult levels. At around birth there is a change in the sensitivity of the liver to exogenous hydrocarbons, and after birth the extent of induction rapidly reaches adult levels. Furthermore, species differences are large and some species like rabbits and guinea pigs are much more resistant to the induction by polycyclic aromatic hydrocarbons than, for example, rat or mouse [63].

Several studies have shown that the placenta does not normally possess
AHH activity. However, exposing a pregnant animal to polycyclic aromatic
hydrocarbons readily induces AHH activity [11]. This ability of placental
AHH to be induced develops gradually from the middle trimester of pregnancy and is highest at term [64].

The human fetus is able to metabolize benzo[a]pyrene [31,65,66] although the level of AHH activity is only a few percent of the adult human
liver level [27,31]. Fetal hepatic AHH is detectable at 6-7 weeks of fetal
age [67] and is apparently not induced by maternal cigarette smoking [68].
On the other hand, the induction of human placental AHH depends heavily on
maternal cigarette smoking [68-70]. In fact, very little activity is present
in the placenta of nonsmoking mothers, whereas maternal cigarette smoking
results in greatly increased activity in most cases, and in heavy smokers
activity approaches that observed in liver.

As just outlined, AHH activity has been used as a probe to study
the general properties of monooxygenase systems in various tissues.
Nebert's group [71] has shown that AHH activity in mouse liver microsomes
can be separated into two entities: (1) "basal hydroxylase activity" associated with cytochrome P-450 in control or phenobarbital-treated animals,
and (2) "aromatic hydrocarbon-inducible hydroxylase activity" associated
with cytochrome P-448 or P-450 in aromatic-hydrocarbon-treated animals.
These forms can be differentiated by preferential inhibitors [72] and by in-
ference from protein patterns following electrophoresis [73]. Figure 2

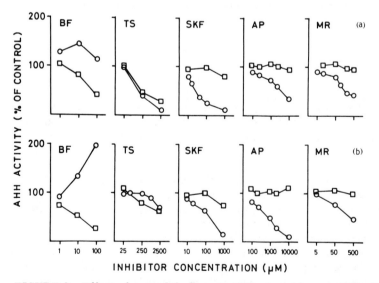

FIGURE 2   Effect of α-naphthoflavone (BF), testosterone (TS), SKF-525A
(SKF), aminopyrine (AP), and metyrapone (MR) on aryl hydrocarbon hydroxylase activity in vitro in human fetal liver and placental homogenates
and rat liver homogenates.

shows the preferential inhibition of human fetal hepatic and placental AHH activities by α-naphthoflavone and other compounds as compared to control and 3-methylcholanthrene-induced rat liver. The differential inhibition of human fetal hepatic AHH by α-naphthoflavone and other compounds classifies it as a P-450-associated hydroxylase, while the corresponding properties of placental AHH designate it as a P-448-associated enzyme [74]. These studies suggested that human fetal hepatic AHH is really "constitutive," and not "induced," by environmental chemical stress, whereas the placental AHH activity reflects the exposure of the mother to environmental polycyclic aromatic hydrocarbons. With respect to animal fetuses, the studies of Welch et al. [75] and Wiebel and Gelboin [76] have shown that AHH activity appearing in the rat fetal and neonatal liver after exposure to polycyclic aromatic hydrocarbons belongs to the class of cytochrome P-448-associated enzymes.

In summary, the human fetus and the fetuses of common laboratory animals also differ with respect to aryl hydrocarbon hydroxylase activity. Livers of animal fetuses are essentially devoid of AHH activity, whereas in the human fetal liver and adrenal glands there is low but significant AHH activity, the properties of which seem to suggest its basal nature. AHH activity is readily inducible in animal fetal tissues and placenta and also in the human placenta by the exposure of the mother to polycyclic aromatic hydrocarbons, whereas the human fetal hepatic enzyme seems to be quite resistant to induction, probably because only low levels of inducers reach the fetal liver.

IV. REGULATION OF EXPRESSION OF DRUG METABOLISM IN THE FETUS AND PLACENTA

A. Induction by Xenobiotics

Drug metabolism in animal fetuses is inducible by the exposure of the mother to various xenobiotics during late pregnancy [19,20; cf. references therein]. In most cases, fetal microsomal enzyme activity can be stimulated only when the inducing compound is administered to the mother during the last few days of gestation. However, some studies indicate that induction may also occur in earlier stages of pregnancy [23,77]. The occurrence of induction seems to depend on the inducer and on the substrate or pathway studied. Generally speaking, cytochrome P-448 inducers like 3-methylcholanthrene, tetrachlorodibenzo-para-dioxine (TCDD), and some polychlorinated biphenyls are the most potent inducers during the perinatal period, whereas phenobarbital or pregnenolone 16α-carbonitrile hardly induce drug metabolism [78-80]. Studies by Guenthner and Mannering [79, 80] further indicate that the simultaneous treatment by phenobarbital and 3-methylcholanthrene induces drug-metabolizing enzymes in the fetal liver to a greater extent than would be expected on the basis of their separate effects. In any case, the extent of induction in fetal liver is always much lower than it is in neonatal or adult liver, and drug-metabolizing enzymes of neonatal animals are more easily inducible than those of fetal animals [81-83], suggesting that the ability to respond to inducing agents increases in the postnatal period.

   With respect to the inducibility of drug-oxidizing systems in the human fetal liver and adrenal glands, much less data are available. Some studies have indicated that xenobiotics (e.g., drugs and alcohol) administered to the mother over a long period and in large doses may induce drug metabolism in human fetal liver during the first half of pregnancy [84]. Studies on the pharmacokinetics of phenytoin [85] and carbamazepine [86] in the newborn human indicate that transplacental induction by these drugs may occur. It thus appears that drug-metabolizing enzymes in human fetal liver are inducible during late pregnancy, while more studies are needed to confirm induction during early pregnancy. Maternal intake of drugs or alcohol has no effect on placental drug-oxidizing enzymes, except in those cases where mothers also occasionally smoked cigarettes [84]. It has been argued that the drug-metabolizing capacity of the human fetus is a consequence of the long-term exposure of the mother to environmental chemical substances. However, this belief may not be correct, at least as far as hepatic and adrenal systems are concerned. The available evidence indicates that the hepatic and adrenal monooxygenase systems are associated with the "basal" form of cytochrome P-450. On the other hand, the placental monooxygenase system metabolizing a few foreign compounds seems to be present in significant amounts only in the placenta of smoking mothers. Thus, the placental system is clearly inducible by environmental factors, and its properties resemble those of the cytochrome P-448-linked system. The apparent noninducibility of the fetal hepatic and adrenal monooxygenase systems does not necessarily mean that they are "intrinsically" noninducible. It may be that in most in vivo situations, the concentration of a potential inducer does not reach the required levels.

B. Effects of Hormones and Inhibitors

Changes in hormonal balance have been suggested to be responsible for the low or absent drug metabolism found in fetuses and may also explain why fetal animals do not respond efficiently to in vivo induction. The hormones thought to be responsible for the suppression of drug metabolism during fetal and neonatal life include progesterone, progesterone metabolites [87, 88], and growth hormone [89]. Although these hormones may be of importance in some situations, the evidence is contradictory [90,91] and a final evaluation is difficult. The most convincing evidence for a role of glucocorticoids in the development of drug-metabolizing enzymes comes from the studies of Wishart and Dutton [92,93]. They suggest that glucocorticoids, which increase in the rat fetus between days 17 and 20 of gestation, trigger

the normal development of hepatic glucuronyltransferase activity toward
ortho-aminophenol. A very interesting study by Manchester and Neims [94]
suggests that the postnatal maturation of hepatic monooxygenase activity
may be a birth-related phenomenon, the mechanism of which is unresolved
but may involve hormonal factors. Also, the gestational age at which this
birth-triggered maturation is acquired, remains unknown.

Several studies have indicated that sex hormones, especially androgens, have a significant role in the development of drug-metabolizing enzymes in young rats [95,96]. Especially interesting in this respect are the
studies of Gustafsson et al. [97] and Tabei and Heinrichs [98] concerning the
neonatal "imprinting" effect of androgens on steroid hydroxylases in rat
tissues. This imprinting also occurs on drug-metabolizing enzymes [99].
Other regulatory factors are implicated, but they are ill defined and their
properties remain unknown; they include fetal inhibitors in liver [100] and
serum [101].

C. Chick Embryo and Fetal Cells as Models of
Mammalian Embryos

Studies with mammalian embryos are complicated by maternal factors.
Mainly to overcome this difficulty, two lines of research have been pursued:
first, the use of avian embryos; and second, the use of organ and cell cultures. Dutton and Burchell [42] have studied the avian embryo, which is
self-sufficient in ovo and amenable to controlable environmental change.
Their studies were mainly focused on UDP-glucuronyltransferase activity
toward xenobiotics and steroids, with some observations on cytochrome
P-450-linked enzyme activities. The activities of drug-metabolizing enzymes
appear to be repressed in ovo, except for a short period between days 12
and 16. They are inducible by phenobarbital injected into eggs. When the
avian embryonic liver is organ-cultured or kept in cell cultures, UDP-glucuronyltransferase activity rises to adult levels or higher, whereas cytochrome P-450-linked enzyme activity disappears [102]. These studies on
avian embryo drug-metabolizing enzymes have also shown remarkable differences when compared with mammalian drug-metabolizing enzymes.
Marked culture-induced increases in UDP-glucuronyltransferase activity
are not seen in mammalian liver; phenobarbital is often unable to induce
this activity, whether in utero or in culture [103]. On the other hand, the
transferase can be prematurely induced by the exposure of fetal rat liver
explants to glucocorticoids [92] or in utero by injecting dexamethasone or
coritsol to the mother [93].

Cells derived from different fetal organs have been extensively used
in the study of the induction of drug-oxidizing enzymes, but the relevance of
this approach with respect to the enzyme regulation in the fetus remains to
be established [104,105].

D. "Intrinsic" Temporal Regulation of Gene Expression

Numerous studies have shown that enzyme activities have distinctive ontogenetic patterns [106], and indeed this is the case for xenobiotic-metabolizing
enzymes (see Sec. II). However, the developmental patterns of drug metabolism may be more complicated than earlier believed, as revealed by
recent investigations. A study by Atlas and collaborators [107] showed that
in the neonatal rabbit, aryl hydrocarbon hydroxylase activity, which in the
adult is not inducible by polycyclic aromatic hydrocarbons, responds to
treatment with 3-methylcholanthrene; this induction is associated with the
appearance of a new gel electrophoretic band in the region of cytochrome
P-450 proteins. Recent studies from the same laboratory [108] show that
a similar kind of perinatal development can also be detected in the rat and
mouse. It thus seems probable that different forms of cytochrome P-450
develop at different times and that the inducibility of these different forms
may also undergo changes during development. Siekevitz [109] has shown
that the gel electrophoretic band corresponding to cytochrome P-450 in rat
liver microsomes is already detectable before birth, although a negligible
drug-oxidizing activity can be detected at that time. This study indicates a
temporal regulation not only for the development of enzyme proteins but
also for the development of functionality in multienzyme systems. It can
be speculated that, when we talk about temporal regulation of the expression
of drug-metabolizing enzymes, we should in fact talk separately about temporal regulation of (1) enzyme proteins, (2) multienzyme systems, and possibly (3) small-molecular-weight modifiers, all of which could be regulated
separately.

E. Implications for the Human Fetus and Placenta

The available evidence indicates that human fetal, neonatal, and placental
drug-metabolizing enzymes are regulated in a manner similar to that in
animals. Fetal hepatic, adrenal, and placental monooxygenase systems
differ from each other [20], while the fetal hepatic system differs from its
adult counterpart in a very specific way, namely, with respect to polycyclic
aromatic hydrocarbon-inducible cytochrome(s) P-450 [74]. Neims et al.
[18] have produced definitive evidence that monooxygenase activity develops
postnatally in a manner depending upon substrate and metabolic pathway.
We can then postulate that different forms of drug-metabolizing enzymes in
human tissues have specific developmental patterns; because we know that
different enzymic forms have different activities and substrate selectivities,
an obvious implication is that the metabolism of foreign compounds at a
given age is both qualitatively and quantitatively different from that at
another age. If we were able to characterize the composition of drug-
metabolizing enzymes at a given age, then we could predict the ability of

an individual to metabolize a wide variety of foreign and endogenous substances. A preliminary attempt in that direction has been made in Table 3,
where the characteristics of fetal and placental enzymes have been differentiated on the basis of postulated forms of cytochrome P-450. Obviously
this scheme is highly hypothetical but may serve as a starting point for
research.

V. PHARMACOLOGICAL AND TOXICOLOGICAL IMPLICATIONS OF FETAL DRUG METABOLISM

A. Steady-State Levels of Xenobiotics

Lack of drug metabolism in the fetus has been regarded as teleologically
meaningful because of the difference assumed to exist in the relative transfer rates of xenobiotics and their metabolites. Indeed, metabolites less
lipid soluble than the parent compound may transfer more slowly back to
the mother and thus accumulate in the fetus. However, the human fetus is
able to metabolize drugs more efficiently than fetuses of other animal species.
   On the basis of the known activity of drug-metabolizing enzymes in
human fetal tissues and placenta and of the theoretical considerations of
Gillette et al. [110] and Gillette and Stripp [111], it is probable that steady-
state levels of foreign compounds in the fetus or in the mother are not ap-
preciably affected by the activity of fetal drug-metabolizing enzymes. Some
exceptions may exist—for example, highly lipid soluble drugs.

B. Accumulation of Metabolites in the Fetus

Theoretically (see Sec. V.A), the significant fetal accumulation of Phase
II metabolites (conjugates) could be expected because they are very water
soluble [for a discussion, see Ref. 20]. The capacity of the human fetus to
conjugate foreign compounds seems to be variable depending on the donor
of the conjugating moiety. Glucuronic acid conjugation appears to become
functional later than oxidative processes. Other conjugates may accumulate
on the fetal side, for example, glycine conjugates, which are probably
readily formed in the human fetal tissues.

C. Xenobiotic-Steroid Interactions

Numerous studies have shown that the human fetal liver, adrenal glands,
and placenta hydroxylate steroids [e.g., 112,113]. Many, perhaps most,
of these steroid hydroxylations are catalyzed by the cytochrome P-450-
linked enzyme systems [see, for example, Ref. 114]. However, it is not
known whether steroid hydroxylases are the same enzymes that hydroxylate
xenobiotic substances.

TABLE 3
Hypothetical Scheme of the Characteristics of the Human Drug–Oxidizing Monooxygenase System

Human tissue	Predominant cytochrome	Molecular weight band		Characteristic catalytic activity	Preferential inhibition
		Rabbit	Rat/mouse		
Fetal liver Adult liver	P–450	50,000	50,000	Benzphetamine N-demethylation	Metyrapone
Placenta Fetal adrenal	P_1–450	57,000	56,000	Aryl hydrocarbon hydroxylase Biphenyl 2-hydroxylase	α–Naphthoflavone
Fetal adrenal	P–448	54,000	54,000	Acetylaminofluorene N-hydroxylase Acetanilide 4-hydroxylase	α–Naphthoflavone

Source: Data from Refs. 73, 74, 107, and 126, as well as the author's unpublished results.

Nothing is known of the possible interference of xenobiotic metabolism with steroid hormone metabolism in the fetus. Interaction between the two have been shown in adult animals and humans [115], and similar interactions may also occur in the human fetus. Their existence, however, remains to be demonstrated.

D. Active Metabolites

The role of active intermediates in the onset of tissue lesions, carcinogenesis and other harmful effects of foreign compounds has received considerable attention during recent years and in a number of cases the relationship between metabolism and toxicity is well established [see, for example, Ref. 116]. The recent study of Sehgal and Hutton [117] showed that rat fetal tissues catalyze the formation of carcinogen metabolites mutagenic to Salmonella typhimurium strains. Pretreatment of pregnant animals with 3-methylcholanthrene increased the catalytic activity. Experimental studies on transplacental carcinogenesis show that agents needing metabolic activation are only effective just before birth when drug-metabolizing enzymes appear in fetal tissues [118]. Studies by Nebert's group have demonstrated an association between teratogenesis and/or fetotoxicity and inducibility of aryl hydrocarbon hydroxylase in inbred strains of mouse [119,120]. All these studies point to the possibility that active intermediates are responsible for some of the harmful effects during fetal life. The ability of the human fetus to oxidize xenobiotics implies that potentially toxic intermediates can be formed [121], and indeed some metabolites have been tentatively proposed as candidates (Table 4). The activity of human fetal enzymes is lower than that of adult enzymes, and thus active intermediates are probably formed in smaller quantities. In this respect, however, the sensitivity of fetal tissues to exogenous influence is important. It is likely that fetal tissues and their functions differ from their adult counterparts with respect to sensitivity to exogenous influences (e.g., xenobiotics and their activated metabolites). The low activity of fetal enzymes does not necessarily mean that there is less likelihood of harmful effects being mediated by their metabolites. In this respect, a few recent findings are of considerable interest. Thus, Blake et al. [122,123] have postulated that the metabolic activation of phenytoin, a possible human teratogen [124], is required to produce its harmful effects. Further, Jones et al. [125] have demonstrated the ability of human fetal tissues and placenta to catalyze the formation of mutagenic metabolites from several carcinogens. The best we can say at this stage is that human fetal tissues are able to activate foreign compounds and thus fulfill one of the prerequisites (but not all) for the production of harmful effects.

TABLE 4
Potential Activation Reactions Catalyzed by in vitro Human Fetal Tissues

Compound	Metabolic pathway	Harmful effects implicated
Benzo[a]pyrene	Epoxidation	Carcinogenesis; mutagenesis
Aldrin	Epoxidation	Increased toxicity
Dimethylnitrosamine	N-Demethylation	Carcinogenesis
Phenytoin	Epoxidation	Teratogenesis (?)
Aniline	N-Oxidation	Methemoglobinemia
2-Acetylaminofluorene	N-Hydroxylation	Carcinogenesis; mutagenesis

Source: Data from Refs. 121, 123, and 125.

VI. CONCLUSION

This brief outline of the development implications of drug metabolism stresses three important points:

1. Temporal regulation of drug metabolism seems to be much more complicated than was believed earlier. It is probable that the emergency and disappearance of different forms of enzymes and even their inducibility may be regulated quite independently, leading to typical and definite patterns of drug metabolism in each species. This area of study is at its beginning stage.

2. Inducibility of drug metabolism during fetal life, although linked to the first point, needs special attention, because changes in our chemical environment may have effects on the delicate balance of numerous enzymes involved in the "detoxification" and "activation" of exogenous and endogenous compounds.

3. Formation of active intermediates by fetal tissues may lead to all the harmful consequences attributed to these "products of teleologically blind enzymes." It may be expected that the few examples already known are only forerunners in the elucidation of the role of harmful intermediates in fetal disfynction and malformations.

blood concentrations and its half-life of elimination. As a consequence, the appearance of the metabolite in urine will be slowed down, even if ultimately the cumulative excretion of the metabolite (P) will be the same in both renal and nonrenal patients.

When metabolism is the rate-limiting step (flip-flop; see Fig. 14), metabolite blood levels may be increased without any modification of the apparent half-life of elimination (flip-flop "$t_{1/2}$") and only limited changes will be observed in the appearance of the metabolite in urine. It is important to recognize that this is not the consequence of a modification of the apparent volume of distribution of the metabolite in the renal patients.

Accumulation of active metabolites can be clinically significant even if the active metabolite is a minor metabolite as long as this molecule is not further biotransformed and is mainly excreted in the urine. The presence of an active metabolite may be important in patients with renal failure for

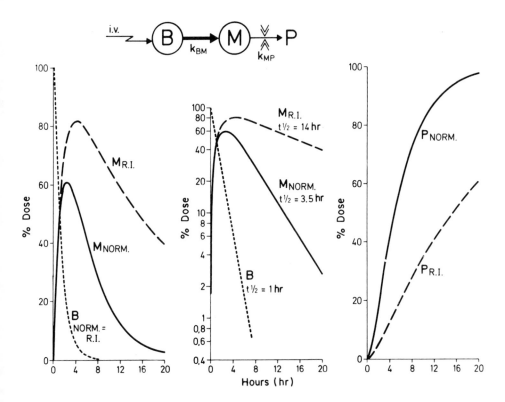

FIGURE 13 Influence of renal insufficiency on the kinetics of a drug and its metabolite when renal excretion of the metabolite is the rate-limiting step.

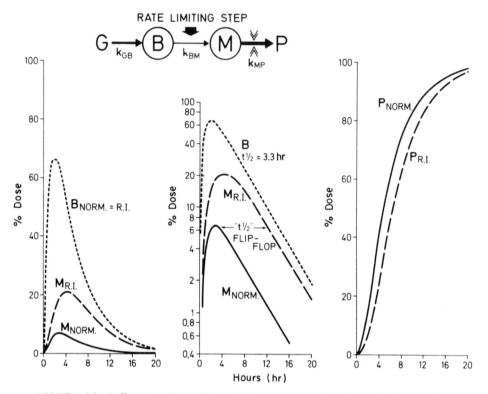

FIGURE 14   Influence of renal insufficiency on the kinetics of a drug and its metabolite when metabolism is the rate-limiting step.

such drugs as procainamide, pethidine, clofibrate, allopurinol, sulfonamides, methyldopa, and nitrofurantoin [51]. It is probable, however, that more drugs will have to be added to this list as more data become available.

For those drugs which are eliminated esséntially by hepatic metabolism or biliary excretion, it is very tempting to assume that patients with renal insufficiency only have a limited capability for the urinary excretion of the metabolite and that all other physiological functions are normal. Unfortunately, patients with renal insufficiency often show modifications of pharmacokinetic parameters that do not bear a direct relationship with the decrease of glomerular filtration rate. Thus, many drugs show alterations of the volume of distribution. For example, edema considerably disturbs the behavior of drugs whose volume of distribution approximately equals the extracellular space, whereas dehydration increases the plasma levels of most drugs.

Many drugs circulate in the blood partly bound to plasma proteins. Abnormal blood protein concentrations, which occur, for example, when the fluid balance is disturbed, make it difficult to predict the likely changes in free plasma drug concentrations. In hypoproteinemia, the unbound levels of drug are higher than under normal conditions. Additionally, functional and anatomical changes to the gastrointestinal tract caused by chronic uremia may affect to some degree the absorption of drugs given orally [50]. All these modifications may alter both the time course of drug metabolism and the kinetic properties of metabolites in renal insufficiency when compared to those observed in patients with normal kidney function.

Indeed, it has been reported that some metabolic pathways may be modified in uremic patients even if other routes of biotransformation appear normal [52]. It is probable that hydroxylation of propranolol is reduced in renal insufficiency [53], and the same findings have been reported for bufuralol [54]. Since for these two drugs metabolism is the only route of elimination of the parent drug and since hydroxylation leads to pharmacologically active metabolites, it is very difficult to predict how renal failure may influence the action of these drugs.

A similar example is shown in Fig. 15. The kinetics of glipizide (a hypoglycemic sulfonylurea) and its main hydroxylated metabolite were studied in normal subjects and in patients with renal insufficiency [44]. If blood and urinary data obtained in normal subjects (Fig. 15a) are treated by compartmental analysis on a computer, it is theoretically possible to predict the behavior of the drug and its main metabolite when their renal handling is modified by kidney dysfunction (Fig. 15b). The computer-predicted behavior of hydroxyglipizide clearly does not reflect the situation found in vivo in a patient with renal insufficiency, even if one corrects for the delayed gastrointestinal absorption observed in the renal patient.

The precise meaning of such findings remain unclear. It must, however, be kept in mind that the kidneys may play an important role in the metabolism of many drugs, as is now well known for vitamin D. We thus feel that the study of the pharmacokinetics of parent drug and metabolites in patients with severe renal insufficiency might greatly improve our understanding of the relative importance of hepatic and renal metabolism, even if these drugs are not designed for chronic use in renal patients.

V. CONCLUSION

It has been shown that, within the limitations of the one-compartment open body model with parallel elimination processes, care has to be taken in the interpretation of the log metabolite concentration versus time curve. In the first instance a highly sensitive, specific analytical technique with frequent data points is necessary to accurately define the shape of the blood concentration versus time curve for metabolites since the terminal segment will be nonlinear when the metabolite elimination rate is similar to its formation rate. As a consequence no half-lives are measureable.

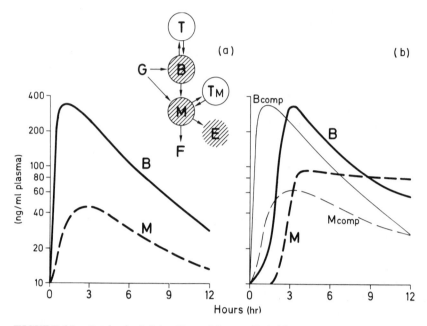

FIGURE 15   Oral administration of 5 mg glipizide to two patients. (a) Plasma concentrations of glipizide (B) and its main hydroxylated metabolite (M) as calculated by compartmental analysis for one subject GFR = 10 ml/min with normal renal function according to a two-compartment open body model for the parent drug and the metabolite. Data is available from the hatched compartments. Symbols: T, peripheral compartment; G, gastrointestinal system; E, renal elimination; F, extrarenal elimination. Glipizide is almost totally metabolized. (b) Computer-simulated plasma concentrations for glipizide (Bcomp) and its main metabolite (Mcomp) taking into account a reduction of the renal function to about one-tenth of its normal value and comparison with data (B and M) obtained in one patient with a GFR of 10 ml/min. The behavior of the parent drug is almost parallel to the predicted values with the exception of a lag time for the gastrointestinal absorption, but metabolite elimination seems much more impaired than its computer-predicted kinetics.

Even when the terminal segment is linear, the half-life measured can be either that of metabolite elimination (when elimination is slower than formation) or that of parent drug elimination (when elimination is faster than formation). The practical consequences of these considerations is that it is difficult to determine the metabolite kinetic parameters when the parent drug has been administered since the elimination of the parent drug and its metabolites do not normally differ by an order of magnitude.

Further consequences of this potential mirror-image or looking-glass behavior in systems with parallel formation processes have been discussed. For example, the pharmacokinetic models usually employed to predict the behavior of drugs subject to first-pass metabolism are inadequate because they do not take into account saturable systems. Consequently, simplified integration routines may lead to wide confidence limits in the estimated pharmacokinetic parameters.

Bioavailability measurements based on metabolite levels will only be correct if the metabolite is pharmacologically active since, when inactive, an overestimate of the bioavailability of the therapeutic moiety may occur. In addition the use of total radioactivity or any other nonspecific assay for this purpose provides only limited information since one can never be sure of the species being measured.

In abnormal situations such as pregnancy and renal insufficiency it is open to question whether dosage regimens should be altered to prevent excessive accumulation of metabolites. However, if these species are potentially toxic of pharmacologically active, we fell alterations should be made.

We have not dealt with the effects that age, sex, genetics, or environmental factors may have on the biotransformation process, but clearly they too must be taken into account when interpreting data. Even if they were considered, we doubt that metabolites would lose their potential to show looking-glass kinetics. We conclude therefore that, practical limitations aside, the only way to accurately elucidate the metabolite pharmacokinetic profile is to administer both metabolite and parent drug in separate experiments.

APPENDIX A: GLOSSARY

1. Symbols Used in the Equations

AUC	Total area under the blood concentration-time curve in the central compartment
B	Amount of parent drug in the central compartment at time t
B(t)	Amount of parent drug in the central compartment as a function of time
$\overline{B}$	Laplace transform of B
b	Parent drug concentration in the central compartment at time t
b_0	Parent drug concentration at time zero
db/dt	Rate of change of parent drug concentration in the central compartment

$\int_0^\infty b\,dt$	Total area under the parent drug concentration in the central compartment versus time curve (AUC)
Cl	Total clearance
$\overline{Cl}_L$	Mean hepatic clearance
$\overline{Cl}_L^{ss}$	Hepatic clearance at steady state
Cl_L	Instantaneous hepatic clearance
$Cl_{L,\,loglin}$	Log linear hepatic clearance
D_0	Dose of parent compound administered at time zero
E	Cumulative amount of parent drug eliminated to time t
F	Fraction of absorbed dose available
F'	Fraction of the administered dose actually absorbed
k_{IJ}	Apparent first-order intercompartmental transfer rate constant for transfer from compartment I to compartment J ("from-into" convention)
K_m	Michaelis constant
K_P	Apparent partition coefficient
M	Amount of metabolite in the central compartment at time t
$\overline{M}$	Laplace transform of M
m	Metabolite concentration in the central compartment at time t
P	Cumulative amount of metabolite eliminated to time t
Q_L	Hepatic blood flow
s	Laplace operator
ss	Steady-state situation
$t_{1/2}$	Apparent half-life of elimination
$"t_{1/2}"$	Flip-flop apparent half-life
V_B	Apparent volume of the central compartment for the parent drug
V_D	Apparent volume of distribution
V_M	Apparent volume of the central compartment for the metabolite
v_{max}	Theoretical maximum rate of process describable by Michaelis-Menten kinetics

2. Useful Definitions

<u>Apparent half-life of elimination</u>: the time required for the drug (or metabolite) concentration at any point during the disposition phase to decrease by one-half.

<u>Apparent volume of the central compartment</u>: proportionality constant relating the concentration of the drug (or metabolites) in the central compartment to the amount present, such as $B = V_B b$.

<u>Apparent volume of distribution</u>: proportionality constant relating the concentration of drug (or metabolite) in the central compartment to the amount of drug (or metabolite) present in the body.

<u>Bioavailability</u>: the measurement of both the relative amount of active principle administered that reaches the general circulation (i.e., the extent of absorption) and the rate at which this occurs.

<u>Biophase</u>: compartment in which the drug receptor sites are located.

<u>Central compartment</u>: the blood and all readily accessible fluids and tissues form the central (or sampling) compartment. It is assumed that any change which occurs in the plasma (or serum) level of a drug quantitatively reflects a change which occurs in central compartment tissue levels.

<u>Clearance</u>: number of milliliters of the volume of distribution "cleared" of drug in a unit time. The total clearance may comprise renal, hepatic, pulmonary, etc., clearances.

<u>Compartment</u>: set of tissues and fluids that may be treated kinetically as a common homogeneous unit. However, kinetic homogeneity does not necessarily mean that the drug concentration is the same in all tissues of the compartment at any given time.

<u>Distribution</u>: act of apportioning or spreading out of a drug in an orderly manner once it reaches the blood circulation.

<u>Elimination phase</u>: portion of the blood concentration versus time curve starting after the drug has been absorbed and distributed. For metabolites it is necessary that all drug has been biotransformed before the elimination phase can be determined or that the metabolite is administered as such in a separate experiment.

<u>Extraction ratio of an organ</u>: fraction of the total content of the blood flow that is extracted by the organ. The extraction ratio (2) relates the clearance to the blood flow such as $Cl = QE$. Blood flow and extraction ratio are independent parameters controlling clearance but, as shown in Appendix D.3, the extraction ratio depends upon blood flow.

First-order kinetics (or linear kinetics): realized when there is a direct proportionality of transfer rates to concentrations or concentration differences between the compartments.

First-pass effect: drug uptake and elimination by the gastrointestinal tract, the liver, or the lungs during the first passage of drug into the circulation after hepatic route administration; it may effectively prevent a significant fraction of the administered dose from reaching the peripheral sampling site.

Flip-flop: kinetic situation occurring when the rate of appearance of a substance (by absorption or formation) is slower than its rate of disappearance.

Hepatic route: oral administration or intraperitoneal, splenic and portal injection. Hepatic routes are contrasted with the peripheral routes such as subcutaneous, intramuscular, or sublingual administration or injection into the femoral, cephalic, or jugular veins.

Lag time: time elapsed between the administration of a drug and its appearance in the circulation, or between its appearance and the manifestation of its biological effect.

Microscopic rate constant: proportionality constant relating the rate of change (dX/dt) to the amount of substance involved, such as $dX/dt = k_{IJ}X$ for the simplest situation.

Model: most commonly employed approach to the pharmacokinetic characterization of a drug by the representation of the body as a system of compartments, even though these compartments often have no apparent physiological or anatomical reality. Models are useful for the description of drug or metabolite time course and for the prediction of the behavior of drugs under conditions not yet studied.

Peripheral compartment: often referred to as tissue compartments; they include all compartments which have different kinetic properties to the central compartment. Usually, the time course of drug levels in a hypothetical peripheral compartment does not exactly correspond to the actual time course of drug levels in any real tissue.

Systemic circulation: in the context of bioavailability, the systemic circulation refers primarily to the venous blood (excluding the hepatic portal blood during the absorption phase) and arterial blood which carries the drug to the tissues.

APPENDIX B: SOME BASIC PHARMACOKINETIC EQUATIONS

1. The One-Compartment Open Body Model with Intravenous Injection

$$\xrightarrow{D_0} \left(B\right) \xrightarrow{k_{BE}} E \qquad \text{SCHEME } 5^*$$

---

*The symbols are defined in Appendix A.1.

Differential equation:

$$\frac{dB}{dt} = -k_{BE}B \quad \text{or} \quad \frac{db}{dt} = -k_{BE}b \tag{28}$$

Integrated form:

$$B(t) = D_0 e^{-k_{BE}t} \quad \text{or} \quad b(t) = \frac{D_0}{V_B} e^{-k_{BE}t} \tag{29}$$

Logarithmic form:

$$\ln B(t) = \ln D_0 - k_{BE}t \quad \text{or} \quad \ln b(t) = \ln \frac{D_0}{V_B} - k_{BE}t \tag{30}$$

The apparent half-life of elimination is defined as:

$$t_{1/2} = \frac{\ln 2}{k_{BE}} \tag{31}$$

Total clearance is defined as:

$$Cl = k_{BE}V_B \tag{32}$$

Dost's law of the corresponding areas may be expressed as:

$$\int_0^\infty b\, dt = AUC = \frac{D_0}{k_{BE}V_B} \tag{33}$$

As a consequence, the area under the concentration versus time curve will be dependent on the administered dose, the elimination rate constant, and the apparent volume of distribution. It does not depend on the rate of appearance of the drug in the body.

It is clear, however, from Eqs. (32) and (33), that if the elimination rate constant is dose-dependent (e.g., saturable elimination) neither the "clearance" nor the "area under the curve" concepts will hold.

The elimination rate of the drug (dE/dt) can be defined as:

$$\frac{dE}{dt} = k_{BE}B \tag{34}$$

Substitution for B, according to Eq. (29) yields:

$$\frac{dE}{dt} = k_{BE}D_0 e^{-k_{BE}t} \tag{35}$$

which, when transformed in its logarithmic form, gives us a straight line:

$$\ln \frac{dE}{dt} = \ln(k_{BE} D_0) - k_{BE} t \tag{36}$$

As a consequence, the drug elimination rate constant (k_{BE}) can be obtained from either blood concentration or urinary excretion data.

In the case of parallel elimination processes, e.g., urinary excretion (E) and metabolism (M), the behavior of the drug can be represented as:

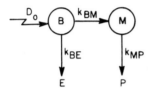

SCHEME 6

Differential equation:

$$\frac{dB}{dt} = -(k_{BE} + k_{BM})B \tag{37}$$

Integrated equation:

$$B(t) = D_0 e^{-(k_{BE} + k_{BM})t} \tag{38}$$

Logarithmic form:

$$\ln B(t) = \ln D_0 - (k_{BE} + k_{BM})t \tag{39}$$

The equations for the apparent elimination half-life, total clearance, and area under the curve are similar to Eqs. (31), (32), and (33), but these parameters are functions of both k_{BE} and k_{BM} such as $t_{1/2} = \ln 2/(k_{BE} + k_{BM})$.

Since, for first-order kinetics, the rate of appearance of unchanged drug in the urine is proportional to the amount of drug in the body, the excretion rate of unchanged drug (dE/dt), can be defined as:

$$\frac{dE}{dt} = k_{BE} B \qquad [\text{Eq. (40)} = \text{Eq. (34)}]$$

Substitution for B, according to Eq. (38), into Eq. (39) yields:

$$\frac{dE}{dt} = k_{BE}D_0 e^{-(k_{BE}+k_{BM})t} \tag{41}$$

which can be written in logarithmic form as:

$$\ln \frac{dE}{dt} = \ln(k_{BE}D_0) - (k_{BE} + k_{BM})t \tag{42}$$

Therefore, a semilogarithmic plot of excretion rate of parent drug versus time is linear, with a slope of $-(k_{BE} + k_{BM})$. This is the same slope as is obtained from blood data for the unchanged drug. It must be emphasized that, in the case of parallel first-order elimination processes, the slope of the logarithm of urinary excretion rate versus time curve is a function of the overall elimination rate constant $(k_{BE} + k_{BM})$, and not of the urinary excretion rate constant (k_{BE}). However if one of the two elimination processes is dose-dependent, none of these equations can be applied [2].

2. The One-Compartment Open Body Model with First-Order Absorption

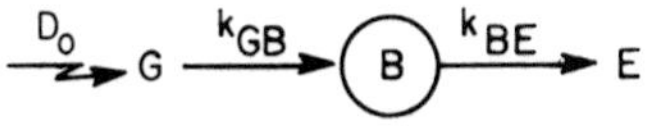

$$\xrightarrow{D_0} G \xrightarrow{k_{GB}} \boxed{B} \xrightarrow{k_{BE}} E$$

SCHEME 7

Differential equation for B:

$$\frac{dB}{dt} = k_{GB}G - k_{BE}B \tag{43}$$

Integrated form:

$$B(t) = D_0 \frac{k_{GB}}{k_{GB} - k_{BE}} \left(e^{-k_{BE}t} - e^{-k_{GB}t} \right) \tag{44}$$

This is the Bateman function (see Sec. I).

The total clearance has the same value as Eq. (32) and, as long as the dose is totally absorbed, the area under the concentration versus time curve is given by Eq. (33). As a consequence, these two parameters are independent of the rate of absorption. Equation (44) is given in terms of "amounts of drug" in the body in function of time; if blood concentrations are considered, it is necessary to divide the dose (D_0) by the apparent volume of distribution of the central compartment (V_B).

As discussed in Sec. I, two cases may occur: $k_{GB} \gg k_{BE}$ (normal situation) and $k_{BE} \gg k_{GB}$ (flip-flop). Great care must be taken in the flip-flop situation not to calculate k_{BE} from the "apparent half-life" since here $t_{1/2} \neq \ln2/k_{BE}$. The same precaution is important for the estimation of the total clearance and the computation of the area under the curve using equations similar to Eqs. (32) or (33) that imply the determination of k_{BE}.

In addition one must distinguish a special case where $k_{GB} = k_{BE} = k'$

Differential form:

$$\frac{dB}{dt} = k'G - k'B \tag{45}$$

Integrated form:

$$B(t) = k'D_0 t e^{-k't} \tag{46}$$

Logarithmic form:

$$\ln B(t) = \ln(k'D_0)t - k't \tag{47}$$

The term $\ln(k'D_0)t$ is responsible for the nonlinearity of the semilogarithmic plot of blood concentrations versus time. As a consequence it is not possible, in this situation, to determine a half-life of elimination.

APPENDIX C: INTEGRATED METABOLITE EQUATIONS FOR INTRAVENOUS INJECTION IN THE ONE-COMPARTMENT OPEN BODY MODEL

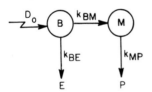

SCHEME 8

1. Normal Situation

Differential equations:

$$\frac{dB}{dt} = - (k_{BE} + k_{BM})B \tag{48}$$

$$\frac{dM}{dt} = k_{BM}B - k_{MP}M \tag{49}$$

Let $\overline{B}$ and $\overline{M}$ be the Laplace transforms of B and M, and s the Laplace operator; then

$$s\overline{B} - D_0 = - (k_{BE} + k_{BM})\overline{B} \tag{50}$$

$$s\overline{M} = k_{BM}\overline{B} - k_{MP}\overline{M} \tag{51}$$

or

$$\overline{B}(s + k_{BE} + k_{BM}) = D_0 \tag{52}$$

$$- \overline{B}k_{BM} + \overline{M}(s + k_{MP}) = 0 \tag{53}$$

Then

$$\begin{bmatrix} (s + k_{BE} + k_{BM}) & 0 \\ -k_{BM} & (s + k_{MP}) \end{bmatrix} \begin{bmatrix} \overline{B} \\ \overline{M} \end{bmatrix} = \begin{bmatrix} D_0 \\ 0 \end{bmatrix} \tag{54}$$

$$\Delta \begin{bmatrix} \overline{B} \\ \overline{M} \end{bmatrix} = \begin{bmatrix} D_0 \\ 0 \end{bmatrix} \tag{55}$$

$$\overline{M} = \frac{\begin{vmatrix} (s + k_{BE} + k_{BM}) & D_0 \\ -k_{BM} & 0 \end{vmatrix}}{\Delta} = \frac{D_0 k_{BM}}{\Delta} \tag{56}$$

by Cramer's rule. But

$$\Delta = \begin{vmatrix} (s + k_{BE} + k_{BM}) & 0 \\ -k_{BM} & (s + k_{MP}) \end{vmatrix} = (s + k_{MP})(s + k_{BE} + k_{BM}) \tag{57}$$

or

$$\Delta = s^2 + s(k_{BE} + k_{BM} + k_{MP}) + k_{MP}(k_{BE} + k_{BM}) \tag{58}$$

$$\Delta = s^2 + s(\alpha + \beta) + \alpha\beta = (s + \alpha)(s + \beta) \tag{59}$$

where

$$\alpha + \beta = (k_{BE} + k_{BM}) + k_{MP} \tag{60}$$

$$\alpha\beta = k_{MP}(k_{BE} + k_{BM}) \tag{61}$$

By substitution of Eq. (59) into (56) one obtains:

$$\overline{M} = \frac{D_0 k_{BM}}{(s + \alpha)(s + \beta)} \tag{62}$$

By Laplace transform one obtains:

$$\frac{M(t)}{D_0} = \frac{k_{BM}}{\beta - \alpha} e^{-\alpha t} - e^{-\beta t} \tag{63}$$

or

$$M(t) = D_0 \frac{k_{BM}}{(k_{BE} + k_{BM}) - k_{MP}} e^{-k_{MP}t} - e^{-(k_{BE}+k_{BM})t} \tag{64}$$

This is the equation which permits the calculation ot the amount of metabolite in the body at any given time after the intravenous administration of the parent drug.

The concentration of the metabolite (m) can be obtained by dividing M(t) by V_M, the apparent volume of distribution of the metabolite.

2. Special Case Where $k_{BM} = k_{MP} = k$ and $k_{BE} = 0$

Differential equations:

$$\frac{dB}{dt} = -kB \tag{65}$$

$$\frac{dM}{dt} = kB - kM \tag{66}$$

Then,

$$s\overline{B} - D_0 = -k\overline{B} \tag{67}$$

$$s\overline{M} = k\overline{B} - k\overline{M} \tag{68}$$

$$\overline{B}(s + k) = D_0$$

$$\overline{Bk} - \overline{M}(k + s) = 0 \tag{70}$$

$$\begin{bmatrix} (s + k) & 0 \\ k & -(k + s) \end{bmatrix} \begin{bmatrix} \overline{B} \\ \overline{M} \end{bmatrix} = \begin{bmatrix} D_0 \\ 0 \end{bmatrix} \tag{71}$$

$$\Delta \begin{bmatrix} \overline{B} \\ \overline{M} \end{bmatrix} = \begin{bmatrix} D_0 \\ 0 \end{bmatrix} \tag{72}$$

$$\overline{M} = \frac{\begin{vmatrix} (s + k) & D_0 \\ k & 0 \end{vmatrix}}{\Delta} = \frac{-D_0 k}{\Delta} \tag{73}$$

$$\Delta = \begin{vmatrix} (s + k) & 0 \\ k & -(s + k) \end{vmatrix} = -(s + k)(s + k) \tag{74}$$

$$\overline{M} = \frac{D_0 K}{(s + k)^2} \quad \text{or} \quad \frac{\overline{M}}{D_0} = \frac{k}{(s + k)^2} \tag{75}$$

Now the Laplace transform of $(As + B)/(s + \overline{A})^2$ is

$$e^{-\overline{A}t}[A + (B - A\overline{A})t]$$

when $A = 0$, this becomes

$$e^{-\overline{A}t}(Bt) = Bte^{-\overline{A}t}$$

i.e.,

$$\frac{M(t)}{D_0} = kte^{-kt} \quad \text{or} \quad M(t) = kD_0 te^{-kt} \tag{76}$$

In its logarithmic form Eq. (76) becomes

$$\ln M(t) = \ln(kD_0) + \ln t - kt \tag{77}$$

which clearly is not the equation of a straight line because of the term $\ln t$.

APPENDIX D: DIFFERENTIAL EQUATIONS FOR SPECIAL MODELS

1. Michaelis-Menten Kinetics

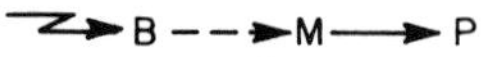

$$\overset{\curvearrowright}{\Rightarrow} B \dashrightarrow M \longrightarrow P$$

SCHEME 9 $\longrightarrow$ first-order kinetics; $- - \rightarrow$ saturable kinetics

$$- \frac{dB}{dt} = \frac{v_{max} B}{K_m + B}$$
differential form   (78)

v_{max} = maximal velocity of the saturable system
K_m = Michaelis-Menten constant (units = concentration)

$$B_0 - B + K_m \ln \frac{B_0}{B} = v_{max} t$$
integrated form, this equation cannot be solved for B   (79)

when $K_m \gg B$

$$- \frac{dB}{dt} \implies \frac{v_{max} B}{K_m}$$
pseudo-first-order elimination for B   (80)

when $B \gg K_m$

$$- \frac{dB}{dt} \implies v_{max}$$
pseudo-zero-order elimination   (80')

If the drug is eliminated in parallel by a saturable and a nonsaturable process, equation 1 becomes:

$$- \frac{dB}{dt} = \frac{v_{max} B}{K_m + B} + k_{ns} B$$
where k_{ns} is the microscopic rate constant for the nonsaturable process   (81)

if $Km \gg B$, Eq. (4) becomes

$$- \frac{dB}{dt} = \left(\frac{v_{max}}{K_m} + k_{ns} \right) B \quad \text{or} \quad - \frac{dB}{dt} = k'B$$
     (82)

where k' is a pseudoapparent rate of first-order elimination.

2. Inhibition of Drug Metabolism

For competitive inhibition, where I is the inhibitor "concentration" and K_I the inhibition constant:

$$- \frac{dB}{dt} = \frac{v_{max} B}{K_m (1 + I/K_I) + B} \tag{83}$$

The application of this equation to predict the kinetics of the interaction necessitates the knowledge of the pharmacokinetic parameters of the drug and its inhibitor, as well as the value of K_I.

3. Hepatic-Blood-Flow-Limited Metabolism

Compartmental analysis is very useful from a descriptive standpoint; however, it bears little direct relationship to the biological factors that control and modify the time course of drug concentrations in the blood or tissues, and this is particularly true for the hepatic or metabolic pathways of drug elimination [53]. Consequently, it is difficult to predict the effects of changes in the biological determinants of drug metabolism, which include the metabolic activity of the liver, its blood flow, and the extent of drug binding to plasma proteins.

Rowland et al. [55] have proposed a "model for perfusion-limited isolated perfused organ systems" which has the clearance (Cl) as key parameter. Here b_L is the concentration of drug in the liver (i.e., the eliminating organ); V_L is the apparent volume of the liver; b_R is the concentration of drug

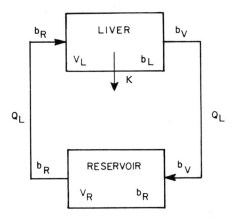

SCHEME 10

in the reservoir (i.e., the sampling compartment); V_R is the apparent volume of the reservoir; b_V is the concentration of drug in the venous blood leaving the liver; Q_L is the blood flow rate entering and leaving the eliminating organ; and k is the first-order rate for drug elimination.

The assumptions are that distribution into the liver is perfusion-rate-limited such that drug in the organ is in equilibrium with that in the emergent venous blood, that the concentration of drug in blood entering the liver equals that in the reservoir (b_R), and that the concentration of blood leaving the liver (b_V) and entering the reservoir are equal.

It is then possible to define a constant $K_P = b_L/b_V$, which is the apparent partition coefficient of drug between the liver and the emergent venous blood; b_0, the initial concentration in the reservoir; and M, the amount of drug eliminated from the system in time t.

Then, when a bolus of drug is introduced into the reservoir (intravenous injection) [see Ref. 5],

$$-V_R \frac{db_R}{dt} = Q_L(b_R - b_V) \tag{84}$$

$$K_P V_L \frac{db_V}{dt} = Q_L(b_R - b_V) - kK_P V_L b_V \tag{85}$$

Solving Eqs. (84) and (85) for b_R and b_V gives Eqs. (86) and (87)

$$b_R(t) = b_0 \left(\frac{(Q_L/K_P V_L) + k - \alpha}{\beta - \alpha} \right) e^{-\alpha t} + b_0 \left(\frac{(Q_L/K_P V_L) + k - \beta}{\alpha - \beta} \right) e^{-\beta t} \tag{86}$$

$$b_V(t) = b_0 \frac{Q_L/K_P V_L}{\beta - \alpha} \left(e^{-\alpha t} - e^{-\beta t} \right) \tag{87}$$

where

$$\alpha + \beta = \frac{Q_L}{K_P V_L} + \frac{Q_L}{V_R} + k \tag{88}$$

and

$$\alpha\beta = \frac{Q_L k}{V_R} \tag{89}$$

The concentration in the reservoir, b_R, declines biexponentially according to Eq. (86). The mean hepatic clearance of drug (the average volume of blood cleared of drug per unit time) $\overline{Cl}_L$ is given by:

$$\overline{Cl}_L = \frac{Dose}{\int_0^\infty b_R \, dt} = \frac{b_0 V_R}{\int_0^\infty b_R \, dt} \tag{90}$$

Since the definite integral of $Ae^{-\alpha t}$ from $t = 0$ to $t = \infty$ is A/α, the total area under the drug concentration in the blood versus time curve after intravenous administration is

$$\int_0^\infty b_R \, dt = \frac{b_0}{\alpha}\left(\frac{(Q_L/K_P V_L) + k - \alpha}{\beta - \alpha}\right) + \frac{b_0}{\beta}\left(\frac{(Q_L/K_P V_L) + k - \beta}{\alpha - \beta}\right) \tag{91}$$

or

$$\int_0^\infty b_R \, dt = b_0 \frac{k + (Q_L/K_P V_L)}{Q_L k/V_R} \tag{92}$$

Substituting Eq. (92) into Eq. (90) yields:

$$\overline{Cl}_L = \frac{Q_L k}{k + (Q_L/K_P V_L)} \tag{93}$$

Equation (93) indicates that the mean hepatic clearance is dependent on blood flow rate (Q_L) and the clearing capacity of the liver as the drug perfuses through the hepatic capillaries.

If, instead of a bolus, drug is infused at a constant rate, k_0, eventually a steady state is approached in which the rate of infusion is balanced by loss of drug; at the steady state the incoming (b_R^{SS}) and outgoing (b_V^{SS}) concentrations remain constant, and it follows from Eqs. (84) and (85) that

$$k_0 = kK_P V_L b_V^{SS} = Q_L (b_R^{SS} - b_V^{SS}) \tag{94}$$

The hepatic clearance at steady state, $\overline{Cl}_L^{SS}$, obtained by measurement across the liver, is given by:

$$\overline{Cl}_L^{SS} = \frac{Q_L (b_R^{SS} - b_V^{SS})}{b_R^{SS}} \tag{95}$$

By substitution from Eq. (94) into Eq. (95) one obtains

$$\overline{Cl}_L^{SS} = kK_P V_L \frac{b_V^{SS}}{b_R^{SS}} = \frac{kK_P V_L Q_L}{kK_P V_L + Q_L} \tag{96}$$

Since Eqs. (93) and (96) are identical, the mean clearance is equal to the steady-state clearance. The fractional term $kK_PV_L/(Q_L + kK_PV_L)$ is termed the extraction ratio of the drug by the liver, while kK_PV_L is the clearing capacity and may be regarded as the maximum volume of blood which could be cleared of drug per unit time were there no flow limitation.

The instantaneous hepatic clearance, Cl_L, is defined by:

$$Cl_L = Q_L \frac{b_R - b_V}{b_R} = Q_L \left(1 - \frac{b_V}{b_R}\right) \tag{97}$$

In the early moments following the intravenous injection of drug the instantaneous clearance is greater than the mean clearance, since the drug simultaneously distributes into the liver and is removed by it. The instantaneous clearance diminishes with time until the ratio b_V/b_R approaches a constant value. Then the instantaneous clearance approaches the so-called log-linear hepatic clearance, $Cl_{L,loglin}$, which is smaller than the steady-state clearance.

If it is assumed that with time $e^{-\alpha t} = 0$, then during the β-phase Eqs. (86) and (87) will approximate to:

$$b_R \Longrightarrow \frac{b_0}{\alpha - \beta} \left(\frac{Q_L}{K_PV_L} + k - \beta\right) e^{-\beta t} \tag{98}$$

$$b_V \Longrightarrow \frac{b_0}{\alpha - \beta} \left(\frac{Q_L}{K_PV_L}\right) e^{-\beta t} \tag{99}$$

then

$$\frac{b_V}{b_R} \Longrightarrow \frac{Q_L}{Q_L + kK_PV_L - \beta K_PV_L} \tag{100}$$

By substituting this value into Eq. (97) one obtains

$$Cl_{L,loglin} = \frac{Q_L K_PV_L(k - \beta)}{Q_L + K_PV_L k - K_PV_L \beta} \tag{101}$$

By suitable substitution from Eqs. (88) and (89) into Eq. (101), the log-linear clearance is found to be

$$Cl_{L,loglin} = V_R \beta \tag{102}$$

Hence, for a given log-linear clearance, β is inversely proportional to the reservoir size. The larger the reservoir size and/or the effective volume of the eliminating organ (i.e., $K_p V_E$), the smaller β becomes relative to k, and the closer the log-linear clearance approaches the steady state clearance.

The concept of clearance can be relatively complex in this application to multicompartmental models. Therefore, a discussion of the influence of distribution characteristics of a drug on body clearance-hepatic elimination relationships is best illustrated employing specific numerical examples as described by Gibaldo and Perrier [2] and Perrier et al. [30]. It can then be demonstrated that the usefulness of biological half-life and body clearance as indices of hepatic elimination are highly dependent upon the pharmacokinetics of the particular drug under consideration. For drugs that confer multicompartmental characteristics on the body, biological half-life is not only a function of elimination but also of tissue distribution; hence, its value as an index of hepatic elimination becomes very questionable. Clearance, on the other hand, is a direct measure of hepatic elimination regardless of the number of compartments conferred upon the body by a drug, provided there is minimal first-pass effect after oral administration.

4. Quantitative Assessment of the Hepatic First-Pass Effect

The essential feature of the models used in this section are that elimination is assumed to occur, at least in part, from a compartment distinct from that containing the vascular sampling site and that this compartment (which is analogous to the hepatoportal system) receives the drug directly upon administration via a hepatic route. For ease of mathematical analysis, only the model shown (Scheme 11) will be analyzed and it is assumed that drug input is instantaneous irrespective of route and that elimination occurs exclusively by metabolism in the liver [2, 28, 29].

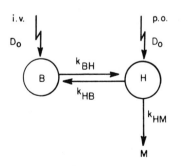

SCHEME 11

Under these conditions, drug levels in compartment B are given by:

$$\frac{dB}{dt} = k_{HB}H - k_{BH}B \tag{103}$$

Since there are two "driving force compartments" in the model, the equation describing the disposition function for compartment B is biexponential and may be written as (for more details, see pharmacokinetic textbooks):

$$B(t)_{i.v.} = \frac{D_0(k_{HB} + k_{HM} - \alpha)}{\beta - \alpha} e^{-\alpha t} + \frac{D_0(k_{HB} + k_{HM} - \beta)}{\alpha - \beta} e^{-\beta t} \tag{104}$$

with

$$\alpha + \beta = k_{BH} + k_{HB} + k_{HM} \tag{105}$$

and

$$\alpha \beta = k_{BH} k_{HM} \tag{106}$$

Converting to concentration terms and rearranging yields:

$$b(t)_{i.v.} = \frac{D_0(k_{HB} + k_{HM} - \alpha)}{V_B(\beta - \alpha)} e^{-\alpha t} - \frac{D_0(k_{HB} + k_{HM} - \beta)}{V_B(\beta - \alpha)} e^{-\beta t} \tag{107}$$

The total area under the drug concentration in blood versus time curve after intravenous administration is given by (cf. Eq. 91)

$$\left(\int_0^\infty b\,dt\right)_{i.v.} = \frac{D_0(k_{HB} + k_{HM} - \alpha)}{\alpha V_B(\beta - \alpha)} - \frac{D_0(k_{HB} + k_{HM} - \beta)}{\beta V_B(\beta - \alpha)} \tag{108}$$

which may be simplified to

$$AUC_{i.v.} = \frac{D_0}{V_B}\left(\frac{k_{HB} + k_{HM}}{k_{BH} k_{HM}}\right) \tag{109}$$

When the drug is administered orally, and assuming instantaneous absorption into compartment H, one obtains the following expression for the amounts of drug in compartment B:

$$B(t)_{p.o.} = \frac{k_{HB}D_0}{\beta - \alpha} e^{-\alpha t} + \frac{k_{HB}D_0}{\alpha - \beta} e^{-\beta t} \tag{110}$$

Converting to concentration terms, and rearranging yields:

$$b(t)_{p.o.} = \frac{k_{HB}D_0}{V_B(\beta - \alpha)} (e^{-\alpha t} - e^{-\beta t}) \tag{111}$$

Integration of Eq. (111) from $t = 0$ to $t = \infty$ yields the total area under the drug concentration in the blood versus time curve after oral administration:

$$AUC_{p.o.} = \frac{D_0}{V_B} \left(\frac{k_{HB}}{k_{BH}k_{HM}} \right) \tag{112}$$

It can be demonstrated that Eqs. (109) and (112) apply regardless of the rate of absorption and of tissue distribution provided that the entire dose is absorbed. The term complete absorption implies that after oral administration the entire dose reaches the portal circulation as intact drug.

Assuming complete absorption, comparison of the areas under the curve after oral and intravenous administration should provide an approach to quantifying the influence of route of administration on drug disposition, at least with respect to the hepatic first-pass effect. Defining the ratio of areas as the systemic availability, F, one finds, if the dose is the same for both routes of administration, that:

$$F = \frac{AUC_{p.o.}}{AUC_{i.v.}} = \frac{k_{HB}}{k_{HB} + k_{HM}} \tag{113}$$

Equation (113) shows that, in theory, the area under the blood drug concentration versus time curve after oral administration will always be less than that observed after intravenous administration if $k_{HM} \neq 0$ and if the volume of distribution is constant. As discussed in Sec. III.A.1, the magnitude of the hepatic first-pass effect can theoretically be estimated from the comparison of k_{HB} and k_{HM}. But since in practice the "liver" cannot be distinguished as a separate compartment, these rate constants cannot be determined and Eq. (113) cannot be solved.

Resolution of this problem is facilitated by introducing certain physiological considerations in the interpretation of the pharmacokinetic model (Scheme 11). Multiplying numerator and denominator of Eq. (113) by the apparent volume of the hepatoportal compartment, V_H, yields:

$$F = \frac{k_{HB}V_H}{k_{HB}V_H + k_{HM}V_H} \tag{114}$$

By assuming that transfer between compartments H and B is blood-flow-rate limited (see Appendix D.3), it can be postulated that:

$$k_{BH}V_B = k_{HB}V_H = Q_L \tag{115}$$

where Q_L is the blood flow rate to the liver. By writing Eq. (115) we postulate that the clearance from one compartment to another is equal in both directions. It follows that:

$$F = \frac{Q_L}{Q_L + k_{HM}V_H} \tag{116}$$

Substituting Eq. (115) into (112) yields:

$$AUC_{p.o.} = \frac{D_0}{k_{HM}V_H} \tag{117}$$

Thus, using Eq. (117) for the evaluation of $k_{HM}V_H$, Eq. (116) yields:

$$F = \frac{Q_L}{Q_L + (D_0/AUC_{p.o.})} \tag{118}$$

If blood level data are available following oral administration of a drug, substitution of the dose D_0 and the total area under the drug level versus time curve, as well as the blood flow rate Q_L (equals about 1.5 liters/min in humans) into Eq. (118) should yield an estimate of F, provided the dose is completely absorbed.

If data obtained after intravenous administration of a drug are available, it is possible to combine Eqs. (113) and (118):

$$F = \frac{AUC_{p.o.}}{AUC_{i.v.}} = \frac{Q_L}{Q_L + (D_0/AUC_{p.o.})} \tag{119}$$

Rearranging yields:

$$F = 1 - \frac{D_0}{Q_L \cdot AUC_{i.v.}} \tag{120}$$

Accordingly, substitution of the intravenous dose and respective total area under the drug level versus time curve as well as the blood flow rate to the liver into Eq. (120) should yield an estimate of the extent to which the first-pass effect contributes to a reduction in the AUC after oral administration relative to that observed after intravenous administration.

If the foregoing approximations and subsequent equations are reasonable, the availability predicted by Eqs. (118) and (120) should agree with that found experimentally. If the actual area ratio is less than predicted, then most likely either absorption after oral administration is incomplete or metabolism occurs in the gastrointestinal tract. If the ratio is greater than predicted, the possibility exists that the concentration of drug in the hepatic portal vein following oral administration may be sufficiently high to saturate the hepatic enzymes. In this case of nonlinear kinetics, the availability of drug to the systemic circulation becomes a function of dose and rate of absorption.

REFERENCES

1. E. R. Garrett, in Klinische Pharmakologie und Pharmakotherapie (H. P. Kuemmerle, E. R. Garrett, and K. H. Spitzi, eds.). Urban & Schwarzenberg, Munich, 1976, pp. 27–52.
2. M. Gibaldi and D. Perrier, Pharmacokinetics. Dekker, New York, 1975, 329 pp.
3. F. H. Dost, Grundlagen der Pharmakokinetik. Thieme, Stuttgart, 1968, 449 pp.
4. J. G. Wagner, Biopharmaceutics and Relevant Pharmacokinetics. Drug Intelligence Publns., Hamilton, Ill., 1971, 375 pp.
5. J. G. Wagner, Fundamentals of Clinical Pharmacokinetics. Drug Intelligence Pubns., Hamilton, Ill., 1975, 461 pp.
6. B. N. La Du, H. G. Mandel, and E. L. Way, Fundamentals of Drug Metabolism and Drug Disposition. Williams & Wilkins, Baltimore, 1971, 615 pp.
7. E. R. Garrett and H. J. Lambert, J. Pharm. Sci. 62:550 (1973).
8. B. Åblad, K. O. Borg, G. Johnsson, C.-G. Regårdh, and L. Sölvell, Life Sci. 14:693 (1974).
9. J. M. Tschopp, A. Gorgia, L. Balant, C. Revillard, R. J. Francis, and J. Fabre, Schweiz. med. Wschr. 108:756 (1978).
10. B. B. Gallagher, I. P. Baumel, and R. H. Mattson, Neurology 22: 1186 (1972).
11. D. L. Smith, T. J. Vecchio, and A. A. Forist, Metabolism 14:229 (1965).
12. L. Hillestad, T. Hansen, and H. Melsom, Clin. Pharmacol. Ther. 16: 485 (1974).
13. U. Klotz, K. H. Antonin, H. Brugel, and P. R. Biek, Clin. Pharmacol. Ther. 21:430 (1977).

14. J. A. Knowles and H. W. Ruelius, Arzneim.-Forsch. 22:687 (1972).
15. L. Balant, J. Fabre, L. Loutan, and H. Samimi, Arzneim.-Forsch. 29: 162 (1979).
16. E. R. Garrett, in Progress Drug Research (E. Jucker, ed.), Vol. 21. Birckhäuser, Basel and Stuttgart, 1977, pp. 105-230.
17. E. R. Garrett, J. Bres, K. Schnelle, and L. L. Rolf, J. Pharmacokin. Biopharm. 2:43 (1974).
18. G. Levy and T. Tsuchiya, N. Engl. J. Med. 287:430 (1972).
19. G. Levy, T. Tsuchiya, and L. P. Amsel, Clin. Pharmacol. Ther. 13: 258 (1972).
20. T. Tsuchiya and G. Levy, J. Pharm. Sci. 61:800 (1972).
21. K. Arnold and N. Gerber, Clin. Pharmacol. Ther. 11:121 (1970).
22. G. W. Houghton and A. Richens, Brit. J. Clin. Pharmacol. 1:155 (1974).
23. A. Richens and A. Dunlop, Lancet ii:247 (1975).
24. M. Rowland, in Drug Metabolism: From Microbe to Man (D. V. Parke and R. L. Smith, eds.). Taylor & Francis, London, 1977, pp. 123-145.
25. M. M. Drucker, S. H. Blondheim, and L. Wislicki, Clin. Sci. 27:133 (1964).
26. P. A. Harris and S. Riegelman, J. Pharm. Sci. 58:71 (1969).
27. R. N. Boyes, H. J. Adams, and B. R. Duce, J. Pharmacol. Exp. Ther. 174:1 (1970).
28. M. Gibaldi and S. Feldman, J. Pharm. Sci. 58:1477 (1969).
29. M. Gibaldi, R. N. Boyes, and S. Feldman, J. Pharm. Sci. 60:1338 (1971).
30. D. Perrier, M. Gibaldi, and R. N. Boyes, J. Pharm. Pharmacol. 25: 256 (1973).
31. E. R. Garrett and C. D. Alway, Proc. 3rd Int. Congr. Chemother., pp. 1666-1686 (1964).
32. L. Balant, Cl. Revillard, and K. Ventouras, Pharm. Acta Helv. 52: 89 (1977).
33. Guidelines for Biopharmaceutical Studies in Man, Academy of Pharmaceutical Sciences, American Pharmaceutical Assn., Washington, D.C., 1972, Appendix I, p. 17.
34. J. P. Skelly, Bioavailability policies and guidelines. Paper presented at the 13th Ann. Int. Ind. Conf. on Lake Travis, Austin, Texas, 1974.
35. C. R. Cleaveland and D. G. Shand, Clin. Pharmacol. Ther. 13:181 (1972).
36. D. G. Shand and R. E. Rangno, Pharmacology 7:159 (1972).
37. B. Åblad, M. Ervik, J. Hallgren, G. Johnsson, and L. Sölvell, Eur. J. Clin. Pharmacol. 5:44 (1972).
38. R. Davies, T. G. Pickering, A. Morganti, G. Bianchetti, P. L. Morselli, J. Romankiewicz, and J. H. Laragh, Lancet i:407 (1978).
39. J. W. Paterson, M. E. Conolly, C. T. Dollery, A. Hayes, and R. G. Cooper, Pharmacol. Clin. 2:127 (1970).

40. J. A. Oates and D. G. Shand, in Biological Effect of Drugs in Relation to Their Plasma Concentrations (D. S. Davies and B. N. C. Prichard, eds.). Macmillan, London, 1973, pp. 97-106.

41. T. Walle, J. Morrison, K. Walle, and E. Conradi, J. Chromatogr. 114:351 (1975).

42. W. J. Westlake, J. Pharm. Sci. 60:882 (1971).

43. B. B. Brodie and J. R. Mitchell, in Biological Effect of Drugs in Relation to Their Plasma Concentrations (D. S. Davies and B. N. C. Prichard, eds.). Macmillan, London, 1973, pp. 1-12.

44. L. Balant, G. Zahnd, A. Gorgia, R. Schwarz, and J. Fabre, Diabetologia 9(Suppl.):331 (1973).

45. L. Balant, J. Fabre, and G. R. Zahnd, Eur. J. Clin. Pharmacol. 8: 63 (1975).

46. B. Krauer and F. Krauer, Clin. Pharmacokin. 2:167 (1977).

47. W. M. Bennett, I. Singer, and C. H. Coggins, J. Amer. Med. Ass. 223:991 (1973).

48. W. L. Chiou and F. H. Hsu, J. Clin. Pharmacol. 15:427 (1975).

49. L. Dettli, Clin. Pharmacokin. 1:126 (1976).

50. J. Fabre and L. Balant, Clin. Pharmacokin. 1:99 (1976).

51. D. E. Drayer, Clin. Pharmacokin. 1:426 (1976).

52. M. M. Reidenberg, Med. Clin. N. Amer. 58:1059 (1974).

53. G. R. Wilkinson and D. G. Shand, Clin. Pharmacol. Ther. 18:377 (1975).

54. L. Balant and T. Tozer, J. Pharmacokin. Biopharm. (in press).

55. M. Rowland, L. Z. Benet, and G. G. Graham, J. Pharmacokin. Biopharm. 1:123 (1973).

Numbers in brackets are reference numbers and indicate that
an author's work is referred to although his name is not cited in
the text. Underlined numbers give the page on which the complete
reference is listed.

Kraychy, S., 7[24], <u>47</u>
Krebs, K. G., 21[59], 22[59], <u>49</u>
Kremers, P., 181[38], 182[38], <u>206</u>
Kriemler, H. P., 215[13], <u>246</u>
Kripalani, K. J., 141[181,182, 183], <u>175</u>
Kristoffersson, J., 66[26], 67[26], <u>170</u>
Krjala, K., 294[45], <u>306</u>
Kuenzig, W., 253[32], 255[32], 260[32], 265[32], <u>280</u>, 288[23], 298[23], <u>306</u>
Kugel, R. B., 229[67], <u>248</u>
Kuhlman, C. F., 36[97], <u>50</u>
Kullberg, M. P., 7[23], <u>47</u>
Kumaki, K., 183[44,46], <u>207</u>, 253[22], 255[22], 260[22], 265[22], 268[22], <u>279</u>, 296[71], 302[126], <u>307</u>, <u>310</u>
Kuntzman, R., 181[33,35,37], <u>206</u>, 270[83,84,86,89,90], 271[83,84, 86,89], 277[84], <u>282</u>, 299[81], <u>308</u>
Küpfer, A., 85[55], 87[55], 122[140], <u>171</u>, <u>174</u>
Kuriyama, S., 24[71], <u>49</u>
Kurtz, W. L., 81[48], <u>170</u>

Labow, R. S., 216[27], <u>246</u>
LaDu, B. N., 178[4], 181[4], <u>205</u>, 253[6,11], <u>279</u>, 315[6], <u>369</u>
Laduron, P., 218[41], <u>247</u>
Laitinen, M., 270[85], <u>282</u>
Lambert, G. H., 274[113], <u>283</u>, 303[119,120], <u>309</u>
Lambert, H. J., 318[7], <u>369</u>
Lan, S. J., 141[182,183], <u>175</u>
Lancaster, R., 237[94], 238[94], <u>249</u>
Landis, W., 200[96], <u>209</u>
Lange, D., 124[150], <u>174</u>
Laragh, J. H., 333[38], <u>370</u>
Larmi, T. K. I., 258[50], 259[50], <u>280</u>, 292[27,36], 296[27], <u>306</u>
Latif, S. A., 253[33], 255[33], <u>280</u>

Lauwers, W. F. J., 84[53], <u>171</u>
Law, F. C., 262-264[72,73], <u>281</u>
Lawson, A. M., 6[17], <u>47</u>
Lawson, P. A., 6[19], <u>47</u>
Layne, D. S., 216[27], <u>246</u>
Leakey, J. E. A., 216[18], <u>246</u>
Leander, K., 101[83.84], <u>172</u>
Lee, E. W., 274[116], <u>283</u>
Lee, M. L., 9[34], <u>48</u>
Lee, Q. H., 287[10], <u>305</u>
Leibman, K. C., 253[7], <u>279</u>
Leighty, E. G., 226[58], <u>248</u>
Leo, A., 148[204], 150[204], 153[204], 155[208], <u>176</u>
Leong, J. L., 277[134], <u>284</u>
Lertratanangkoon, K., 6[13], 42[13,123], <u>47</u>, <u>57</u>
Leutz, J. C., 260[67,68], <u>281</u>
Levin, W., 113[121], <u>173</u>, 180[14, 19,20], 181[33,35,37,40], <u>206</u>, <u>207</u>, 274[117,118], <u>283</u>, 291[24], 295[63], <u>306</u>, <u>307</u>
Levitt, R. C., 274[113], <u>283</u>
Levy, A., 80[45,46], <u>170</u>
Levy, G., 79[43], <u>170</u>, 218[36,38], 236, 237[97,98,101], 238[90, 97,98], <u>247</u>, <u>249</u>, 325[18,19, 20], <u>370</u>
Levy, G. C., 25[79], <u>49</u>
Leuvy, G. A., 294[39], <u>306</u>
Lewellen, O. R. W., 232[80], <u>248</u>
Lewi, P. J., 84[54], 85[54], <u>171</u>
Lewis, R. J., 201[101], <u>209</u>
Li, Y., 4[4], 6[4], <u>47</u>
Lichtenberger, F., 106[101], <u>172</u>, 186[60], <u>208</u>
Lien, E. J., 144[200], 148[204], 150[204], 153[204], <u>176</u>
Lin, C., 4[4], 6[4], <u>47</u>
Lindeke, B., 103[92], <u>172</u>
Linder, R. E., 106[103], <u>172</u>
Lindgren, J.-E., 41[117], <u>51</u>, 101[84,86], <u>172</u>
Linnett, J. W., 194[77], <u>208</u>